I BELONG
FROM CANCER TO WHOLENESS

BIANCA LEPORI

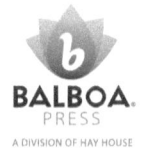

BALBOA
PRESS

A DIVISION OF HAY HOUSE

Balboa Press books may be ordered through booksellers or by contacting:

Balboa Press
A Division of Hay House
1663 Liberty Drive
Bloomington, IN 47403
www.balboapress.com
1-(877) 407-4847

ISBN: 978-1-4525-5889-9 (sc)
ISBN : 978-1-4525-5887-5 (hc)
ISBN: 978-1-4525-5888-2 (e)

Library of Congress Control Number: 2012917159

Printed in the United States of America

Balboa Press rev. date: 11/19/2012

To all visible and invisible helpers

and

to Tobias Giorgia and Martina

CONTENTS

Acknowledgements ix

Preface xi

Introduction xv

Prologue xxi

Chapter 1: Lost in cancer: investigating physiology 1

Chapter 2: Rebuilding the immune system and facing
mastectomy: listening to my spiritual guide
and to myself 17

Chapter 3: Mind, emotions and cancer: learning from
Neuroscience the biochemistry of the
unconscious mind 34

Chapter 4: Vitamin C injections and auric healing:
experimenting with the reationship between
physical and energetic bodies. 50

Chapter 5: Remission and back again: Learning from
Finances and failing as utopian entrepreneur 58

Chapter 6: What am I doing here? Losing ability to
conform and learning from shamanism 70

Chapter 7: Tiferet, the place of Beauty between earth and
sky: remembering Kabbalah 84

Chapter 8: The spreading of the disease: going deeper
into healing by learning from previous lives 101

Chapter 9: Chemically removing the last resistances to
life: chemotherapy as redeemer 114

Epilogue and the Unveiling of the Karmic knot 123

ACKNOWLEDGEMENTS

I N THE STRUGGLE TO face cancer in an unorthodox way I sought the advice and help of a number of people. I should thank in particular Gabriella dall'Acqua for her generous support of my choice in the first phases of the disease, Shirley van Velden for equally nursing my weakness and unorthodox behaviour and Anna Maria Beltrame for accompanying me with her openness into any possible attempt to find personalised ways of healing myself.

I am indebted to Hertha Koettner Smith for her rigorous critique directing me towards restructuring the book into its present shape. I also thank her for her patient dedication in editing the preface, introduction and prologue.

I am profoundly grateful to Chrisjean Tiberti for her empathic concern and offer to help me with the editing of all chapters and for her mindful partnership, careful reading, diligent and participatory revision of the entire manuscript. I also thank Christa Trenz Brower as well as Gabriella dall'Acqua again for their comments on my first writing material and helpful discussions leading to the final draft.

I want to thank Liliana Schiavoni who clarified for me the need to be present to the present and who encouraged me to complete the manuscript and Nunzia Meskalila Coppola who threw light on my original wound and firmly pointed how the publishing of this work would open the doors to my future.

This book would not have been possible without all those who contributed to my healing and prefer to be anonymous. To them my immeasurable gratitude.

My thankfulness also to those who could not understand my way of dealing with the disease but did not comment on it and kept silent, despite their fear and concern for my life.

A special thank you to Balboa press for supporting 'our author within'.

PREFACE

THIS BOOK IS THE autobiographical report of a journey through breast cancer experienced as an opportunity to heal, both the physical and the non physical parts of myself. More specifically it illustrates the long process through which a soul in torment has come to gracefully reconnect with its essential purity and timelessness.

As stated in the title and the subtitle, its purpose is twofold: to demonstrate how the call of an illness can be experienced as a process of re-appropriation of one's own original nature and purpose within the one of the universe; and, as underlined by the subtitle, to specifically share the pilgrimage of progressive defoliation started with the cancer diagnosis, in a cleansing process of initiation to wholeness.

The central threads, portraying an experience rather than a theory, are the non casualness of the disease and the continuum each existence belongs to within the cosmic process of evolution of consciousness. Because of these main themes, involving esoteric disciplines and a subjective experience related to specific body-mind relations, and despite their unfitness to be officially accepted as evidence by traditional science, the book intends to challenge the conventional Western mechanistic medical approaches, and the ones to cancer specifically,unquestionably partial in relation to their frames of reference involving primarily physical matter and, in the better cases, psychological issues contextualized within the current life's events.

Being at first the expression of my own initial intuition, then of a grasping and finally of the embodied awareness of belonging to a continuity in evolution, the content of this work develops through phases in accordance with the pace of my understanding. It progressively introduces the holistic knowledge of ancient eastern techniques and beliefs as well as complementary medicine, homeopathy, psychosomatics, neuroscience, shamanism, and eventually reincarnation as expression of the possibilities for the soul to evolve, according to karmic astrology and quantum physics.

While expressing strong believes as a result of the healing process, the subject questions cultural indoctrination as the two previous books I respectively wrote and co-authored as architect, one on 'Birth Places' and one on 'Architecture from the Inside Out' : the former enquiring about the ergonomics of Medicalized environments for physiological birth and proposing new layouts allowing freedom of movement for women, the latter challenging abstract ways of designing by pointing out, with the support of a technique called Space Therapy, the needs of people's three bodies: the moving, the feeling and the dreaming ones.

By dealing with the healing of design, from the point of view of the physical body and primarily of body and psyche respectively, these two publications, expressing my own need to comply to the roles of honoured conventional scientific theses, have been laying the foundation of this specific work, which represents their further transmutation by manifesting what in them was an implicit necessity. In the attempt to heal my body rather than the design of physical surroundings, thus by going personal rather than being concerned with objectified realities, I allow myself, therefore this book, to go beyond the constrains of accepted verifiable parameters and introduce the spiritual, as universal layout containing all possible design choices.

Avoiding conditioned responses and privileging conscious individual choices, as I have been practising and 'preaching' in my professional work, become therefore here the opportunity of walking firstly my desires and then my talk and, by moving blindly from the inside out through the process, redesign myself and have a glimpse of life design.

In the experience I want to share I hope that the reader may find further tools to open up to her/his own source and nature and become aware of being in a universe engaged, like each of us, in becoming aware of itself.

I am deeply indebted to all scholars and visionaries who have contributed to the perspective of this book, in particular Thorwald Dethlefsen for his work on disease and its relationship with previous lives, Aidin Steinstalz and Z'ev ben Shimon Halevi for their enlightening explanations of the structure of the universe and the journey of descent and ascent of the soul, according to Kabbalah tradition; Peter Russel for his insight into the evolution of Consciousness and Ian Stevenson for his research on reincarnation as a continuation of a particular consciousness; Michael Newton for his clinical soul memories research; Lynn Mc Taggart for the information shared through her magazine What Doctors Don't Tell You and for her experiments on intention and the living field; Barbara Brennan for her studies on the human energy field; Candace Perth for her ground breaking research in neuroscience about the body mind relationship and Deepack Chopra for his contribution to holistic medicine; Amit Goswami for his book Physics of the Soul.

INTRODUCTION

FOR MEDICAL STATISTICS THERE is nothing unique about each individual case of breast cancer since 1.1 million women are diagnosed with it throughout the world every year. However, as a matter of fact, the single case, representing for the medical records an infinitesimal anonymous fraction, is for each woman the whole, her own and specific case, individually experienced according to her nature.

This book is about this uniqueness and the choice, after the diagnosis of a malignant carcinoma, of taking to the extreme consequences personal beliefs and existential questioning. Thus it is about going my own way by listening to myself without relying on the recommended standard medical protocols.

More specifically the choice is based, in the first place, on the assumption that the tumour is not a simple mechanical issue. It is then founded on the underlying query about the threefold question: who am I, where do I come from, what am I here to do and, ultimately, on the hypothesis that cancer is an opportunity to both give evidence of my beliefs and deepen, if not answer, my basic existential questions.

There I was indeed: on one hand I could leave my body, thus I would have taken the short cut towards knowing, but lost the chance of this incarnation; on the other I could experiment, through the messages of my body, the coherence of my beliefs in psychosomatics and stretch them to the very end where the healing of the cause would eliminate the symptoms. I did not have a family to be accountable for, nor a stable partner, nor a child, thus I was free to take the risk and be my own case study, the guinea pig of my solitary un-sponsored searching.

It has been indeed a matter of life or death, in relation to both, my body and my search of meaning on this earth and beyond it. An incredible challenge. I could not just believe, I needed to be scientific about my beliefs, I needed to test them on myself and this could have happened only outside all theoretical worlds, including the one of orthodox western science.

By providing a way of looking at and understanding the slow process of unwinding in conjunction with the different phases of the disease, examined over a period of 14 years, and by reporting related outcomes, the book's intention is to build a case study of what I have experienced with an inquisitive attitude. This in order to generate hypotheses stretching its uniqueness and individuality, if not into generally applicable criteria, into suggestions and possibilities.

The subject of the case study inquiry is a joint venture with breast cancer. A process-journey in which the missing and the unknown are the underlying issue of the desperate searching drive of a person who cannot remember but knows of a quality of being and giving she can never be up to as if prevented by a program she equally ignores. Within the process, at first the tumour is experienced as a matter of negligence on my part, a behavioural impasse and a mere physiological issue. Progressively it is perceived as the screaming of my soul, as the expression of the alliance between body and soul in order to threaten my utmost stubborn self, with something as extreme as death and corner me to the point of making me unable to escape my true responsibility. This is specifically faced in the last phase by entering deep emotional wounds pertaining to previous lives. The physical disease at this point becomes irrelevant, leaving full stage to the inescapable task towards the healing of the soul requiring the coming to the end of the lives-long conflictual obstinate necessity to run away from what needed to be faced in order to be dissolved.

My story portrays the complexity of the energetic levels involved in disease, more specifically the multi faced regions crossed along the journey such as specific therapeutic approaches applied to a physical body and progressively to subtler bodies and energetic levels in order to meet the needs of an ancient consciousness increasingly less unaware of itself.

Nothing of what I am going to say in the book is new: all symptoms have already been analysed in their meaning and catalogued accordingly. Breast cancer specifically has been exhaustively analysed by Rudiger Dahlke (1) in his book Disease As Language of the Soul, where he offers a deep insight into the causes of such a type of tumour, quoting, between these a 'neglected femininity' which is absolutely applicable even in my case. The journey described here lingers on these avenues as well, wondering about which aspect of the feminine I have ignored, but also what Femininity was specifically asking me to express and which aspect of Femininity I was not expressing and why. The multi-layered non-straightforward answers, including the crucial 'because', revealed itself as coming from far away, from within the biography of the original sparkle incarnated in my body. From what I have until recently thought was the CV carried by the soul on its path of descent together with the draft of a business plan of ascent and that I now feel belonging instead to its direction-less and yet structured and purposefully flowing cosmic path.

Although the journey has been characterized by my gropingly moving in darkness, it follows a systematic inner map, which will be adopted in the book as guideline. The mass and the variety of information related to the complexity and articulation of the experience will be framed into three phases: a mainly pragmatical one firstly, secondly an existential one and thirdly a more specifically spiritual one.

The first phase starts with the shock of the diagnosis and is concerned with how I faced the 3.5 cm infiltrating carcinoma physiologically with simultaneous psychological considerations and meditation. The former, in order to boost a debilitated immune system, and bringing back the body's defences that seemed to be lacking, the latter to modify specific behavioural patterns.

Lasting one year, this phase ended with energetic healing, which left me feeling triumphantly recovered; unaware that I had only made a first step in the right direction and that the symptoms would return in order to give me more elements to work with towards the quest.

The second phase, deals with the relapse seven years after remission and is focused mainly on containing the disease, while getting accustomed both to it and to my failure of understanding its deep cause. It includes as broad entry the idealistic and passionate professional time leading to a downside slide. From the point of view of the healing, it is the most difficult phase because, all along, I am also cornered with financial matters, thus I am unable to buy the external help I might have benefited from as in the first phase. It is a time in which I am feeling very much at a loss; the intellect surrendering and withdrawing from the world of action. Almost a spectator, I am existentially an outsider, at the edge of society where everything seams nonsensical while at the same time I am progressively more and more convinced of being unable to heal myself from within.

Forced to free myself from any worldly needs and in isolation, I am in essence like the tarot 'hanged man' with goods falling off his upside down pockets, but preparing himself to enter its archetypal opposite, the tightrope walker.

Third and last phase, emerging from the previous unconventionally ascetic one, tells about the sudden acknowledgement, the need to raise my own level of awareness, moving from all possible alternative and complementary methods I have been involved with, to the essence of my inner life, the spark of light, my inner treasure and leads to the unpredictable dissolution of my true dis-easiness and pain and to the recollection and reconnection with a loving nature and an all embracing universe.

The three phases are further divided into chapters. To explain their reasons within the frame of a life preparing, and asking for all this to happen, a prologue will introduce them.

An epilogue will close the experience from a new life perspective.

The book is not characterized by a consistent writing style. This varies through the script according to the journey scenarios and atmosphere, thus to the moods experienced or the information given. The first chapter, in particular, is characterized by a direct and tense emotional voice, particularly intense in the monologues and inner conversations with "C", as I used to call my joint venture partner.

Bibliography

1 – Rudiger Dahlke – http://www.netplaces.com/spells-charms/
   health-spells/emotional-patterns-and-health.htm

PROLOGUE

A DOPTED FROM THE GREEK tragedy, whose play was introduced by a prologue revealing the events prior to its action, this section briefly informs you, the reader, about the personal context antecedent the cancer diagnosis and adventure.

To be fair to the lesson of the experience, thus to its teaching, leading back to a specific previous life in Renaissance times, the prologue should concern those specific circumstances. Being unveiled at the end of the process, these are instead described in the epilogue, while, in order to be coherent with the original blindness I had approached the disease with, the context that will introduce the action here is not the one pertaining to an ancient drama of my soul but to the one of a personality or ego fully involved professionally in social and ethical issues, bridges on which she has been indulging before being thrust towards the more specific directions described in this work.

In 1988 I realized that Birth Places, and delivery rooms in particular, were inadequate to support women's needs: by analysing the way they were designed I detected that 100% of them were planned to suit the needs of the medical practitioner, not the woman giving birth. Their layout was underlying the intention of intervening upon birth, thus of interfering with the natural process acted by mother and child.

Having found from statistics that only a small percentage of births are complicated, thus in need of intervention, and that the number of these increases because of the inappropriateness of protocols supported by environment, furniture types and layout, I felt the need to professionally unveil the 'misunderstanding'.

Convinced that a change was absolutely essential, I started to travel around the world to wherever I could find and share information that would help me formulate and justify it. I participated in conferences on home birth, natural birth, midwifery, visited the most authoritative people in the field, in Europe and USA, and listened to and interviewed women, anthropologists, midwives, psychologists and doctors. By blending the collected data with my interest in the human psyche and the effects upon this by the environment, I started to envisage which exactly were the changes that needed to be introduced in the birth environment in order to allow the process to unfold naturally.

By interviewing women who had given birth at home I learned that they never expose themselves at the centre of the scene, but instead choose an empty protected area. Rather than a bedroom, they choose a sitting room in which, their feet solidly on the floor, they kneel and crouch between furniture and choose other postures that relax the pelvic floor and allow gravity to help birth take place.

My first and immediate understanding was that a true woman-centred perspective in birth places had to dispose of the dominant position of the bed in the childbirth room. This alone would have given women more options for finding the positions best suited to them for their labour and delivery. (1)

I subsequently learned that the semi supine position, imposed by most obstetricians, obstructs and complicates delivery: it produces the lowest contraction efficiency, increases maternal discomfort and reduces the amount of blood reaching the placenta, thus increasing breathing difficulty for the child. In addition, the necessary internal rotation of the baby within the pelvic canal becomes more difficult and painful for the woman when she is kept in a fixed position on the delivery bed. Furthermore, in contrast, when a woman is free to move around the delivery room to find her own, more comfortable positions, she experiences less anxiety and pain, more efficient contractions, shorter labour and better cardiopulmonary functioning during delivery.

This collection of data was enough to challenge at least, if not change, the *status quo*, (2) and this is what I did. I concentrated the above information in a book-manual and started to stimulate the cultural change in conjunction with professionals of the physiology of birth. Out of the 'preaching' came the commission for a few experimental projects in public hospitals in Italy. The new design consisted of a room in which the woman could move around freely and change position whenever she wished. The bed (that had become a platform) was moved away from the centre, various means of support scattered throughout the room, such as bars, low parapets, towels hanging from the ceiling, a movable birthing stool and a pool.

Through a holistic approach to childbirth, by focusing on woman and child as a whole, my projects had aspired towards reintegrating the birth experience, and consequently the value of birth places, dismissed by contemporary 'one-sided' medicalisation. Had my obsession been with the one-sided medicalisation because I had always felt its inability to heal the wound of my soul even when I was not aware of having been injured at all? While the logical subtitle for my work's task those days was :'The end of the Cartesian mind in birth practice and environment' I was nevertheless using my own mind to sponsor the split between emotions and reason.

In accordance with the Changing Childbirth initiative, (3) started in 1993 in the United Kingdom and with the report of the Changing Childbirth Expert Maternity Group, for which I have been a consultant, my work was based on the assumption that the avoidance of physical death was only the first step towards women's satisfaction at birth. It was suggesting how, despite its focus on 'saving physical life', the medical way was utterly denying women bodily needs, let alone its interference with the chemical and biological reactions related to their emotional state and cultural values making of a 'delivery' 'a life experience'. The one I was not interested in having, physically, but which, I came to discover, had actually been unforgettable for my soul.

My care and my true concern were nevertheless for the new born baby.

The interest in the topic had been awakened specifically by my niece's eyes staring and talking to me, in full consciousness, from her cradle in the nursery a few hours after her birth.

The absolute broad awareness of those grey eyes made it compulsory for me to enter the birth and perinatal field. Something very profound had clicked at that moment and, coherently with my attitude to build intellectual structures tangent in a focal point to the roundness of the emotions, with the tools and the professional credibility I had as architect, I followed an urge that I interpreted as the one of dignifying the environment for the royalty of a soul coming to earth.

> *Our birth is but a sleep and a forgetting;*
> *The Soul that rises with us, our life's star,*
> *Hath had elsewhere Its setting*
> *And cometh from afar."* (4)

Convinced of the full presence at birth of the new 'energetic being', but ignoring the needs of my own energetic being, I went off on a tangent and started searching, interviewing, and designing prototypes of birth places that were celebrating birth from the new born perspective.

I was so generically protective towards them and passionately advocating for their comfort and well being! The welcoming reassuring atmosphere I cared so much to promote, soon shifted to the perfect place for a physiological birth in support of the symbiotic relationship between mother and child. Feeling the sacredness of that bond I had even enquired into the animal realm almost to justify the feline rage against mother and child separation after birth.

Then, in support of women's freedom of movement at birth I entered the market place, and paid a dear price for this, mainly because it was handled predominantly by male doctors, corporation managers and product salesmen.

I was keeping a high cultural quality profile, but, besides ignoring the reasons of my soul, I was muddying my own intention at a level that was lower and profane, according to the high spiritual standard I thought I was motivated by, and moving from. Yes, I had indeed introduced into my practice and teachings, the concept of designing for people's three bodies: the one that moves, the one that feels and the one that dreams. But I never dared to explicitly mention what I cared so much about and what I was sure to be made of: the bodies of light.

By ignoring this, let alone the urging of my soul, I was at least betraying my ethics and myself.

Bibliography

1 – http://www.dh.gov.uk/en/Publicationsandstatistics/ Publications/PublicationsPolicyAndGuidance/DH_4005211

2 – *Status quo*, a commonly used form of the original Latin "status quo" – literally "the state in which" – is a Latin term meaning the current or existing state of affairs. To maintain the status quo is to keep the things the way they presently are. http://en.wikipedia.org/wiki/Status_quo

3 – Children Environment 11/2/1994 Bianca Lepori Freedom of Movement in Birth Places http://www.colorado.edu/ journals/cye/11_2/11_2article1.pdf

4 – Intimations of Immortality, Wordsworth. From Frank Homer Curtiss – Reincarnations – Willing Publishing Company San Gabriel California 1949 – page 9

CHAPTER 1

LOST IN CANCER: INVESTIGATING PHYSIOLOGY

A LIFE OF PROJECTS and so many agendas: a type a stereotype an archetype a prototype of change. A lonely, desperate way of being, loved, may be, of giving, expressing, creating through matter.

Ethics and Art an urgency of the soul. Samaritan at the well, pouring out clear water and soiling herself with mud in the process, wasted in a commercial and greedy world. There, as a virgin whore, I positioned myself with a split heart of unspoken intentions, preaching coherence but avoiding the practice.

Continuously confusing general purpose with task, mission with emotion, the essence with its form, I ran from the spring to the greedy rather than thirsty ones, losing both the jar and the well and I went home with empty hands, having been robbed along the way, misinterpreted, misunderstood, misplaced. Strong, starving successfully advocating, sharing.

Too early, too soon, too alone.

Investments in projects, in my learning, in promotions from which others would benefit. Imagining nevertheless to be able, feeling like flying absolutely above, running on the harsh hills of Aulides, (1) unaware of hunters and danger; of wolves, sharks, blood, sacrificial altars, violence, abuse, killing. Are we not just sisters after all?

"Brother, what did you say, you said yes, cancer, it must be cancer, biopsy soon?" And I was standing there, meagre against a wall. Grey trousers, white shirt and a purple Luisa Spagnoli jersey, top of a far too serious twin set. A very very ordinary start, a *'deus ex machina'* *(2)* Doctor and a Patient, an anonymous protocol.

Your fear their fear, their inability to be human, to humanize. Ignorance more than detachment or, possibly, routine. "What shall I eat?" my only question. "No red meat". "I am vegetarian". "Come back in two days for results".

I knew it was you. I knew I had created you despite diets, holistic awareness and psychic notions. *I was* convinced of the specific motivations and healing power of illness, as explained in Thorwald Dethlefsen's (3) books I was introduced to by his scholar and Translator, dear Eva, the beautiful, Venusian Austrian Aphrodite, now ghosting away, consumed by a second visit of breast cancer. I was also intrigued by the idea that disease did not affect Egyptian initiates because of their pure connection to the source, as explained by Paul Brunton in *A Search in Secret Egypt (4)*.

I wasn't ready for you. Can one ever be ready for you? Still I have been carrying with me Lawrence LeShan's *You can fight for your life (5)*, subtitled, I remember, *Emotional Factors in the Treatment of Cancer*, bought subsequently to my visit to Rose in Chichester. The handsome Cathedral and the walk after lunch through the fields. Blackcurrants and her activity then, a counsellor accompanying dying patients; her comments about that particular woman, I don't remember who she was, "who became ill immediately after retirement and departing within three months". I had literally carried the book from country to country without reading it, always on the verge of doing so.

It was there, just in case, or rather as an affirmation to cling to.

And then there was the Gerson therapy, which (6) I always thought I would have chosen, in case I should need to face a cancer diagnosis.

The way I had understood it, it made a lot of sense to me; a natural detoxifying diet, a soft way to reintegrate the body with all sorts of vitamins and minerals from the juice of fresh organic vegetables and fruits. Coffee enemas to eliminate toxins from the colon and liver; a way to cleanse and regenerate oneself through nature.

While carrying a book based on psychological principles pertaining to cancer I knew I would have adopted a method based on the theory that disease is caused by the body's accumulation of toxic substances. A pragmatic approach that made a lot of sense, favoured by fresh fruits and vegetables, which were my preferred food.

The biopsy report read: "Infiltrating carcinoma of the breast" and the doctor said "You will immediately start chemotherapy in order to reduce the 3.5 cm lump before removing it. Call me Saturday morning after 10.30 and I will dictate the list of all the required preliminary exams.

"There is no point in operating to remove just one part", was the contextual message from my spiritual guide as reported over the telephone by the channel in Turin: "Your cancer has spread all through your body".

Indeed I was fading, falling on the stairs at the office. I remember Cecilia bringing chocolate bars to my desk in order to cheer me up and give me energy. Sweet Cecilia. She did not know, neither did I at the time, that chocolate was not something to eat when you are around, as it feeds you, which is not exactly a very good idea. I went for the Gerson Therapy immediately and bought a flight to London, where Maria Claudia was the expert, swami yoga teacher, great mother, colleague and dear friend. She had used the method to heal her own arthritis.

I left Rome just after having made the phone call to the doctor who instructed me about the list of blood tests. I took notes about each while standing on the platform at the Anagnina bus station, waiting for the coach that would take me to Ciampino airport. No cheap Ryanair flights in those days.

That first night I stayed in the Sloane Square area, a guest of Susan, who honoured me, by offering as sleeping room the 'ivory tower', her sanctuary for healing treatments. This cosy, peaceful loft space, next to her top floor apartment, had been cleared of the mythic and dusty stored crafted works and fabrics of her previous activity as a textile dealer.

A cure for all cancers (7) caught my eye, title on a blue cover I had noticed while climbing the ladder to the mezzanine bed. I grabbed that gift from the universe but did not read much because it was very hard for my mind to concentrate. I only gave it a cursory glance, enough to detect a hint of hope, to understand that there was a great deal ahead to discover. The author was Dr. Hulda Clark.

Lying down in that soft, silent, calming, creamy white paradise I could not get away from the underlying unformulated question: "Who was, who is, who started this?" nor from the compulsory answer "I, the strong, the weak the weakest, Me" Between tears and hope and further questions about the "why me"? "why us" ?, while wondering whether you would leave me, for ever, for good or never, I held you for the first time. I felt the warmth of my right palm on your hot pulsating mass and imagined your response. I sensed that we were in touch, perceiving each other and I started to talk to your cells gone mad, scattered like my way of living. I was indeed a destructive cancer cell gone mad out of carelessness: just as your cells did not stop dividing when they should and indeed kept multiplying, I continued being proactive without being able to come to a standstill for a time of reflection and recollection.

I could almost see your cells and I remember talking to them too, asking for forgiveness. "Do please, please reverse your pattern. I promise, I do promise, I will change mine first. Please please please please forgive me, I wasn't aware, calm down please I will look after myself. Do please, do please stop growing inconsiderately, slow down your growth, I wasn't aware, I wasn't".

Across the Thames, from Chelsea to Brixton, the following day Maria Claudia immediately started with the cleansing of my body. She said the Gerson Therapy was far too complicated as it required daily drinking of juice from approximately 20 pounds of freshly crushed organic fruits and vegetables.

One had to think of all the travelling to find them, plus the cost, not to mention the various supplements and treatment recommended as part of the cure. It was becoming obvious that, to follow it through methodically and hopefully successfully, I had to book a place in a US clinic, an option even more unaffordable than the diet.

"We shall practice *Pawanmuktasana*" she said, as if I knew about the asana sequences she was so familiar with. In order to purify all organs the practice was to include internal and external cleansing. "We shall start with the *Jala Neti*, the nasal cleansing therapy. More precisely with the most simple technique consisting in inserting the cone of special tea pot like utensil filled with slightly salty water into one nostril and let the water flow out of the other nostril". Out in her rear garden, among the blue periwinkles, squatting as in an Indian ashram, I was initiated.

According to her, breathing was also crucial, and she put me and my exhaustion and lack of energy into any possible exercise of consciously breathing in and out. Addressing the underlying imbalance, causing the disease, rather than treating the symptoms, Maria Claudia also put me on a strict macrobiotic diet while handing out selected papers, addresses, brochures, products and book reviews. Among them, *What doctors don't tell you (8)*, a magazine whose articles clarified my sensations and justified them.

No more feelings but science, physiology. All this was happening at incredible speed while my 'guruesse' was consistently pointing out the need of eliminating toxins in order to enhance the immune function, while I was trying to find something. I still did not know what it could be. There was one certainty, though, and that was that body cleansing and detoxifying could have offered an inappropriate terrain for cancer and contrast its growth.

We were experimenting, better still she was implementing and supporting me in my experimenting. Soon we placed an order for two bottles of Essiac Original Formula (9) of Rene Caisse, the new product from Canada, advertised as powerful against cancer. It was certainly a boosting blend for the immune system thanks to the nature of the four organic herbs (burdock root, slipper elm bark, sheep sorrel and turkey rhubarb root) it contained. I did not see any of the results I was expecting, at least not the ones I was eager to see on the opaque grey of my face nor in the dimensions of the lump. No other changes either.

What could I have expected after all from two bottles of syrup?

I was ready to trust anything, to give any sign I received a chance. I did not want chemotherapy or an operation. This was becoming increasingly clear. I needed to care for what I had neglected. I could not damage my body any further.

I was hoping for a way, but no way could be found, all alternatives were considered complementary to the surgical removal of the malignant lump and were applicable only afterwards. The malignancy. Were you malignant or simply desperate? What about me who had created you? Nobody was even considering the possibility of a transformation of the mass, a sort of calming down and domestication of the panther. "Get rid of the lump first, then you can try anything" was the answer from Centres and Clinics I had contacted with hope.

I went to Oxford to meet Claire, an acquaintance from the birthing research, a woman from the complementary medical field whose experience and suggestions I valued highly.She had just had her lump removed and was advocating in favour of mistletoe, the vine used for Christmas decorations, as a cure, and against *Tamoxiphen*, that was just a new name to me. It was interesting to discover another type of cure based on plants. I was feeling generally very sympathetic toward Mistletoe, which by the way is poisonous, but was offered for treatment under the label, *Iscador* (10), the filtered extract made from grinding the entire plant after it had been soaked and fermented in water.

Claire explained the interesting twofold function of *Iscador*: that of feeding the weakened immune system cells, thus preventing the rise of cancer and their growth as well as the one of acting directly on the malignant cancer cells. Potentially poisonous, *Iscador* was administrated by injections of progressively more concentrated extract. This therapy was well supported by Rodolph Steiner's followers because of its integration of the physical and spiritual components. I became intrigued by this.

"Watch out for *Tamoxiphen*", Claire added, handling a paper with evidence from recent research. *Tamoxiphen* was the largest selling drug for the treatment of breast cancer. For reasons I did not grasp, it could contribute to reducing cancer and be carcinogenic at the same time. In particular, the paper stated how it was proven that the incidence of ovarian cysts and cancer was increased when *Tamoxiphen* had been used as a cure for breast cancer. Therefore no *Tamoxiphen* during the radio or chemotherapy stages, nor after it, she recommended. Was I going to go through that? Hopefully not, but, how could I have sustained my point of view with all supporters of a medical approach, with all doctors colleagues and friends I had been and I was working with, aiming to get rid of the lump first? Mistletoe seemed to be an option, something that might have worked, but surely not a solution, nor a method with certified results.

Was there a guaranteed result? The only certainty was my conviction to reduce the damage rather than increase it. My way of keeping the promise of my night in the ivory tower was going to be pursued thanks to the signs with which I was progressively presented. I was becoming aware of both the immune system working in favour of eliminating carcinogenic cells and of the free radicals working in favour of them. My entire body needed to know that I was becoming conscious of this dichotomy. Thus, from that moment onwards, I would be careful and my cells, all of them, the wise ones and those that had gone crazy, would physically perceive the change in the way I would nourish them.

The immune system. Why hadn't I been informed about it at school for instance? Why had there been no classes on health and disease prevention? Why had no doctor ever even mentioned this to me or to my mother when I was a child, or to my friends; the ones who died, the ones who have survived? Did anybody know? Might it have been that, for any precise reasons, the proper functioning of the body was concealed as I had learned was the case with the physiology of birth?

For decades I had been a follower of Abraham Maslow (11), the Humanistic Psychologist and his mind blowing revolutionary point of view. With a focus on self-actualized people he had analysed the mentally healthy individuals rather than the ones with pathological issues and, as a consequence, he had believed that in every person there is a drive to be in harmony physically and physiologically with oneself and one's surroundings. Permeated by his positive approach I was aiming to explore a similar humanistic one in Medicine, with the intention of analysing how healthy bodies would function.

Maslow assumed that each of us has inner resources for healing and that the purpose of psychological therapies is to contribute to removing the obstacles preventing this from happening. Focusing on positive natural functioning was so much healthier than working on pathology which increasingly stirred up more. The analogy was very powerful. Why not focus on the healthy body, on the physiological chemistry of its healthy functioning rather than work on mending the consequent pathology? A positive approach that would not contribute to keeping alive and profitable certain professions, exasperating inadequateness, guilt and suffocating people with the negativity of an overwhelming purposely fabricated system. A way that would challenge the generalized tendency to surrender to the priests in white, brokers between lay people and the abstract Science's Eternal Father.

I remember reading that our body is a citadel in which the immune system defends us against attacks by unwanted invaders. According to the sources of those days of mine in London, cancer could develop when the immune system was debilitated or malfunctioning. Repairing and enhancing the immune system seemed to be the key towards health and, in my case, healing.

I decided then to work on my citadel, my field, and bring back all the right conditions in order for the immune cells to recognize their role again and be in charge of defence. My understanding in simple terms was that it was a matter of boosting the immune system. 'Boosting' a new very effective word, to make its cells strong enough to consume the unwanted ones. Between the six basic types of cells able to respond to foreign attacks and eliminate them, the most powerful were called T cells (12), the ones that seamed suitable to also fight cancer cells. Where had my T cells gone? What had I done to them? Were they on strike because of the low wages leading them to malnutrition? Why wasn't I striking then instead of saving on my food in order to cope with the expenses of office, rent and practice for the sake of carrying out solitary commitments fundamentally towards my beliefs? T cells were not serving their enemy, as instead I was. They were simply not serving me anymore, quite rightly, I thought. I needed to do the same and decided to stop working for a while by going on voluntary, solitary strike. I definitely sympathized with and learned from them. They had been reduced to a condition of weakness that had made them unable to fully perform their role and respond to the insubordination generated from within my citadel.

I also became aware of the chemical nature of my field. Images from school and diagrams came about with electrons and protons, nucleus, atoms, all elements composing a cell. In a normally functioning field, the immune system would contribute to keeping its stability. Stability, I had understood, was generated by stable bonds between atoms with an even number of electrons. When bonds were characterized by the presence of an odd number of electrons in the atoms, stability was threatened because of the unstable bonds producing unstable fields.

Meanwhile I was learning that free radicals, born out of the splitting of weak bonds between electrons, had an uneven number of electrons, thus, by trying to achieve stability they were looking for their missing electron in the near-by atoms, stealing the electron, so to speak, and leaving unstable in its own turn the atom, that would have done the same. This chain reaction would have weakened molecule after molecule and cancer cells would be created.

Instability in my life too. Was I a free radical then? Was there a connection between this and my feeling very radical and frequently incurring in the epithet of 'free spirit' ? Was I missing a bond or was I purposely deciding not to connect? Even when in deep constant conflict with a strongly structured *status quo*, radical people are not necessarily dangerous for its stability and may not even be a threat to a powerfully dominating intolerable system. The *status quo* may indeed be very incompatible, uncomfortable, suffocating and deadly damaging for a free spirit's powerless passion rather than vice versa. Thus the metaphor of free spirits and free radicals does not seam applicable.

How to stop the cascading process then? Who could have been the subject capable of doing so and bringing back the system into balance?

Antioxidants, I was learning, were the generous characters in the arena, almost detached heroes, Round Table's Knights, programmed advocates of justice, goodness and mercy. So prosperous and generous, so much above dichotomies, they played the role of helping the weakest by donating one of their own electrons in order to stop the electron stealing reaction. I was discovering not to have enough antioxidants in my body, thus not enough chivalrous knights fighting for its well being. I certainly needed to reintegrate them.

The introduction of poisonous chemotherapy attackers onto the uprising cancer cells as well as onto the not carcinogenic ones in a body already invaded by free radicals and with not enough antioxidants definitely did not make sense. Chemical attackers seemed irrational in the humanistic economy of my health and I was progressively feeling more strongly that my way should have been the one of weakening the pathogenic attackers in my body by chemically strengthening the generous potential of local heroes. There was no need to drop bombs over my simple shaky shelters.

There was already a fight going on and the only way I could envisage facing it was by relying on the body's ability to heal itself without further negative side effects.

In support of all this I discovered information about a conference on *An Alternative Cure for Cancer (13)* organized by the *What Doctors Don't Tell You* magazine and held in London in 1996, the year prior my diagnosis. Quite a twist of fate, I thought, since tapes were available. I immediately called the indicated Editorial number and off I went to their premises in Islington. Of the four tapes I bought, I mostly resonated with Dr. Kingsley's (14) presentation, because he gave voice to my beliefs by adding and blending information and crucial revelations to which I started to adhere. I took plenty of notes from his ground-breaking lecture contributing to further knowledge about physiology and its chemistry, about what to and not do and why in order not to unbalance my system any further but rather bring it back into balance.

With all the above I became unwaveringly aware that one is not 'hit by cancer' as is commonly said in Italy. Cancer does develop for certain reasons, thus it can be thwarted by mending its causes. It was a matter of strengthening the positive in order to weaken the negative and thus change the relationship between the elements as in the Einstein formula $E=mc2$, which states that any form of energy can be transformed into another form with 'E' remaining unchanged.

The key points of Dr Kinglsey's therapy were the boosting of the immune system, the monitoring of free radicals and the use of antioxidants, vitamin C in particular, the awareness of the anaerobic nature of cancer cells and the support of homeopathy in counteracting the chemotherapy treatment's side effects. Quite enough food for thought as well as, being a Torus Aquarius ascendant, for action.

Whereas normal body cells meet their energy needs by oxygenation, Kingsley explained that cancer cells meet their energy needs mainly by fermentation. An excellent example of what doctors don't tell you, but, I was wondering, do they know this at all? Are all Hospital designers aware of this when building air conditioned, often windowless, day hospital wards for oncology patients? The fantastic news was that cancer cannot exist in oxygenated cells thus, by increasing the levels of this chemical element in them, an environment is created where cancer cannot easily survive.

Dr Kingsley's recommended diet was consisting in avoiding wheat, yeast, refined carbohydrates, dairy products, coffee and in eating fresh fruits and vegetable, cauliflowers and broccoli in particular. Indeed I came to appreciate even more the no sugar, no yeast diktat of Maria Claudia and smiled to her perseverance in checking my breathing exercises, all aiming to stop you growing and to suffocate you with lots of oxygen.

Consequent to the exposed principles deduced from physiology, the Kingsley protocol consisted of high doses, of ascorbic acid or vitamin C, at least 10 grams per day, and hydrogen peroxide taken intravenously. As antioxidant, the former was assumed to protect all but the cancer cells from oxidative free radical damage, and the latter was firing the cancer cells and the equally anaerobic free radicals. As a consequence I took conscious breathing as a must.

With the help of homeopathic remedies Kingsley also brought relief to people undergoing chemotherapy. He suggested that Ainsworth (15) the well known homeopathic chemist in London, not far from the Wighmore concert Hall, could provide safe and non-toxic remedies tailored to each one's chemotherapy. These would prevent its side effects without diminishing the intended effects of the toxic treatment used to cure a disease produced by an already far too weak and intoxicated body.

The conference speeches were very much from the point of view of supporting the body and that specific Kingsley tape was a manifestation of humility. I listened to the wisdom of the organic system stated as a matter-of-fact.

Scientific knowledge away from the experimental practices of indiscriminately bombarding the whole body with poison, too simplistic and paradoxically naïve despite their sophisticated names labels and formulas.

No, I would not accept any chemotherapy, I could not do this to my already suffering body, I did not want to hurt billions in the hope of getting rid of the millions of you. You, the imbalance I had created. You the terrifying terrorist, the unpredictably devastating you. You needed to be loved, so did I. You could not love, I could.

Amaroli (16) was also mentioned as a cure. With fantastic skin, Maria Claudia herself was promoting its use and made me realize that, after completing the cleansing, I could also approach that therapy, the Indian practice, consisting of drinking one's own urine. (17)

Sickening enough for our western taste, urine chemically contains the cleansed substances distilled from the eaten food, whose toxic components are carried through the digestive tube and colon. In other words, as Maria Claudia explained, by drinking it, one would reintegrate the body with what it was missing. A macrobiotic diet including raw food was essential. Proteins and sugar needed instead to be avoided.

Sufficiently disgusted by the idea I came to terms with its naturalness, as compared once again to *farmaka,* the synthetic poisons of the corporations. "If I am so much against the latter I could be in favour of the former, couldn't I?"

Maria Claudia's partner and also a colleague, had just been on a TV program about amaroli. What was so absurdly repellent about that liquid containing mainly vitamins and salt since, as I was learning, all toxins were going into the solid stuff? Possibly the area it was coming from? Why should it be a necessarily revolting experience?

Was I detoxified enough to be safe in trying? Was I ready to trust the body and be prepared to drink that, I had understood, was not the discharged thus contaminated, polluted and smelly release as I had always considered it ?

It was with a full champagne glass that I toasted with Maria Claudia and her partner to the decision of trusting the inner ability of the body to rebalance itself. Nothing disgusting about the golden liquid: the taste was slightly salty, it could have been a drink made out of a mineral solution.

If I could drink this, I told myself, I could trust the process of doing everything from within. The choice was made: to nourish myself so positively to the point of having you surrender and dissolve out of too much goodness and delight. I was dreaming of a trend reversal, a back warding process towards your dissolution and absorption. Would this have been possible? I was feeling it or at least I was sure that this could have been my only way.

From Dr. Clark, and her book *A cure for all cancer* Maria Claudia was further exploring the so called "zapping" she already knew about. I had neither time nor energy for that since I was concentrated on trying to make sense and doing everything according to my beliefs, often while still in the process of discovering them. I was aware of acknowledging them sometimes prior to their rational formulation as if I was believing even prior to uncovering beliefs.

The so called Zappers, where the therapeutic tools emitting electromagnetic impulses aiming to fire at bacteria or parasites through the zapping process. They were indeed precious tools contributing to the cleansing of the body, but I could not think of bacteria and parasites as well. Toxins were more than enough. I already had so much to handle, too much to deal with, including the uncertainty about you in the background. I was unwinding my entire mind set not to mention my life set-up. So I dedicated myself to detoxifying my system despite Maria Claudia interest in eliminating my parasites as well and in building a zapper, which I was not ready for, so determined was I with sticking to my intentions, the actual way to manifest them still to be found. There was also a cacophony about the name of the tool and something disgusting about the idea of parasites. Where could they have been?

For some reason the sound of the name and this further uncertainty were producing rejection and more anxiety than the cancer itself, a further concern with ugly resonances, a thought I could not handle.

Maria Claudia was also pointing out the need to avoid computer radiation, which I promised to keep at a distance. Appalled by the chemical products I was using to dye my hair with, she more than once mentioned the need of coming to an end with that habit too. I was not ready, psychologically, to change my appearance as well.

Bibliography

1 – Euripides -Iphygenia in Aulides - Aulides, town from which, according to the myth, the Achaean fleet sailed off to Troy. In its surroundings Iphygenia, Agamemnon daughter, is sacrificed to Arthemis in order for the winds to calm down and allow the fleet to set off.

2 – Something or someone that comes in the nick of time to solve a difficulty, especially in works of fiction. This Latin term is a translation from the original Greek and owes its origin to Greek drama. '*Deus ex machina*', literally '*god from the machina*' refers to the machina - the device by which gods were suspended above the stage in the Greek theatre. This began being used in English texts from around the middle of the 17th century. http://www.phrases.org.uk/meanings/deus-ex-machina.html

3 – Rudiger Dahlke, Thorwald Dethlefsen – The healing power of illness: the healing of symptoms and how to interpret them - Element Books Ltd 1974 –

4 – Paul Brunton- A search in secret Egypt – Weiser Books; Revised edition December 1984

5 – Lawrence Le Shan – You can fight for your life – Emotional factors in the treatment of cancer M.Evans & Company (February 15, 1980)

6 – A Cancer Therapy: Results of Fifty Cases and the Cure of Advanced Cancer by Max Gerson and Charlotte Gerson (Paperback - 1958) Gerson Institute, 6th edition (1958)

7 – A cure for all cancers – Houlda Regehr Clark. New Century Press (June 6, 1993)

8 – What Doctors Don't Tell You- http://www.wddry.com

9 – Essiac Original Formula – Renè Caisse: www.essiacproducts. com

10 – Iscador : www.iscador.com

11 – Abraham Maslow Towards a Psychology of being: Second Edition (Mass Market Paperback -1968)

12 – T cells or T lymphocites belong to a group of white blood cells known as lymphocites and play a central role in cell-mediated immunity.
http://en.wikipedia.org/wiki/T_cell

13 – Conference : An Alternative Cure for Cancer. What doctor don't tell you. London 1996

14 – Dr. Patrick Kingsley- www.cancer-choices.com

15 – Ainsworths Homeopathic Pharmacy- London – www.ainsworths.com

16 – Amaroli Dr. Swami Shankardevananda Saraswati, Swami Satyananda Saraswati and Dr. Swami Vivekananda Saraswati (Paperback -Dec 1978) Bihar School of Yoga, India (December 1978)

17 – Urine-Therapy It may save your life dr Beatrice Bartnett Lifestyle Institute Margate, Fla

CHAPTER 2

REBUILDING THE IMMUNE SYSTEM AND FACING MASTECTOMY: LISTENING TO MY SPIRITUAL GUIDE AND TO MYSELF

A FTER THREE WEEKS OF a crash course on the physiology of cancer, my time in London had expired and I returned to Italy pre set for home made *chapaties;* deep breathing and a diet consisting of two strict lists, the "yes" one with red beetroot and seitan among others and the "no" one with yeast, fried food, sugar, wine and beer, canned food, cappuccino and *cornetto.*

Except for The Gerson Therapy and for the Dr. Kinsgley's method, I had not found in the UK any institution that could have fully brought forward or supported a way that would be alternative to the orthodox one. Was there at all any means of bypassing the canonical approach and, if so, anyone I could afford? Finances were motivating my decisions. Gerson and Kingsley had been primarily excluded because of their cost. Was I confused? Where was I going? How would I have practically handled the reality of you?

Although the refusal of the medical approach had its justifications, I could not see any alternative that could be systematically adopted. Furthermore, the complexity I was facing was indicating that, despite my determination, I could not continue on my own. The unavoidable questions were becoming even more shocking than the disease : what have I done, what is wrong with my beliefs, feelings and behaviours? I could not just try to overcome the physical disease without grasping the dis-easiness that had motivated it.

I knew too well about the *Unbearable Image* (1) so simply described in Raphael Lopez-Pedraza's article, published in 'Spring', a Journal of Archetype and Culture which made so much sense to me.

Our mind, according to the author, an analytical and archetypal psychologist, can cope with difficulties, conflicts or dislikes and assist us in behaving as if these things did not exist or at least in believing that, rationally, they are a bearable issue. However, Lopez-Pedraza reported that these elements build up an unconscious discomfort that could eventually become a psychic image, emotionally no longer bearable thus manifesting in the body expressing the person's "un-easiness" in the form of a "dis-ease".

Being utterly in tune with it, I was drawn towards the compulsory need to understand where I was unauthentic and what I had been self-imposing if not inflicting on myself. What had I been ignoring to the point of creating such a vexation as reaction?

Having embraced the captivating and convincing theory, I could not but believe that the body would take over psychic suffering and spell it out through physical symptoms that needed to be interpreted or de-constructed in order to face, not so much the cause of the disease, as the dis-easiness producing it. By simply speaking a cryptic and painful truth, the body function was the one of manifesting the need for an existential shift from performing to being. A very arduous reorganization of the mind's controlling skill into an acknowledging ability, requiring a resetting of is monitoring activity. This necessitated absolute protection from unwanted intrusions. A twofold task was therefore at hand: a conscious ending of the manipulation of the unacceptable into something welcomed and satisfactory and also the taking on of the illness by the methods of cure I would select.

The orthodox process would not be suitable, both for the intoxicating destructive approach and for the unavoidable giving in to doctors and professors who would become responsible for my body's life while not accountable for its death. That would have been the consequence of this type of disease or, as it had been proven to be for my father, of heart failure, as if his heart had been the engine of an ordinary auto-mobile.

That would have been far too simple and what would have been the point of being cured without knowing the true, not yet diagnosed pathology which was the source of the disease? I could not see a reason for living apparently 'repaired' without having removed the unbearable image, which, by remaining hidden, would have eventually sprung out as disease again after the removal of the lump. I was in the process of co-writing the book *Architecture Inside Out (2)* about architecture faced from the users' perspective and about buildings and environments seen as energy fields rather than as simple combinations of matter and materials. Was there going to happen some big inside out in me as well? Was I possibly an inside out addict wanting to apply a similar approach to the healing of myself as well?

Acquisition accumulated in the UK were technicalities that needed to be applied in Italy where I was also planning to find out about the symptoms causes. The information I had gained allowed me to find a constructive way to frame the problem physiologically and to strengthen my responsibility towards my own health. As for the unbearable image I had grasped, it had something to do with the feminine and with a mislaid way of giving. I was looking forward to the channelled meeting I had already booked with my spiritual guide since, only through that, would I start to enter the existential reasons behind the physiological evidence.

While waiting for the day of the coming together with my spiritual guide through the medium, I was wondering whom I could have approached in Rome with a sympathetic if not like-minded attitude. I was alone with cancer without wanting to cure it as doctors were suggesting and as everybody was doing and expecting. Who would have supported this unusual, border line and, for some, suicidal approach without fearing it, without asking questions, analysing it, or breaking it into pieces, or slamming directly a door on my face without even listening? I was secretive and very cautious and circumspect in revealing the diagnosis, as if I had to protect the non orthodox approach just as I would have done with a clandestine conspiracy.

Was there somebody who might embrace the entire package of my choice including the unpredictability of result, let alone the method I had not even found as yet ? As sure enough there was no method yet. I was simply facing the process of softly walking in darkness, moving lightly without even knowing the type of ground I was walking on. Not even resting on stepping stones, representing a propulsive spring to move away from rather than a safe place to land. The concern was where to go next by just trusting signs. It was like being in a forest, alone, as I had been so many times, when, as a child, I would run away in the woods surrounding our home.

"Little Bianca is off to the woods", my colleague and dear friend Mark used to say when I was not there, with my mind, presence or attention. Literally running away into the woods had always been my inclination when I wanted to avoid contradictions and useless questions. Thus, metaphorically doing so in similar circumstances was almost inevitable, the crucial difference being that the former had the connotation of immersing myself and re-emerging into a calm and all embracing well known and friendly natural surroundings, the latter of trusting darkness in an unfamiliar environment.

I had met Veronica that same year, a few months before the diagnosis, at a numerology seminar. She was a many-sided psychoanalyst, like I was a multifaceted architect and, like me, interested, as I soon discovered, in finding a terrace with an apartment. A perfect enough ground to sympathize for somebody like myself, always ready to understand peoples' nature from the house of their dreams. In the name of these interests I had visited her once after the conference by limping to her flat with a swollen injured ankle after having fallen off the stairs at the office due to weakness. To my joy I had not only walked away from our meeting painless, loose and recovered by a few simple touches of her hands, but also intrigued and full of curiosity for her vivacious mind, broad culture, creativity and interest in snooping into any achievable psychic or scientific breakthrough; let alone music and graphology that I discovered were among her passions.

"Could I say?" I was wondering "Could she hold the weight and the responsibility of knowing, even more, could she understand the choice?"

Those were the questions running through my mind while sitting in front of her for the second time in her apartment. "My husband died of brain cancer", she said after hearing of my diagnosis," Unfortunately we came across alternative approaches only at a late stage".

Without having to tell her more about the uncertain path I had chosen, she immediately mentioned somebody whom, according to her, I might want to see: a couple living not far from Rome, a lady biologist and her husband.

I have always acted out of faith and the source I had always been drawing from, without carefully listening to, as if resting on my laurels, was now becoming a collection of signs I was attentively and wildly listening to, like an animal smelling tracks leading back home. The "Woman of coincidences", as I had been addressed in the title of a poem in the early eighties, was becoming very serious about the gifts she was offered, honouring them as the only available light. More than coincidences, ciphers, precise messages in code becoming the stepping stones on which to move.

During that same meeting Veronica mentioned the Simontons (3), Carl and his wife, specifically dealing with the topic of fighting for one's life through visualisation, in a tiny book she immediately showed and lent to me. There was something tender about that publication. The story was about a child focusing on his tumour and imagining a pink mouse biting it until it actually dissolved, almost as in a fairy tale. "I will quietly try with you", I whispered softly in my mind and started to practice on that same day.

Soon I was also able to see on the computer screen of the biologist indicated by Veronica, the enlargement of a drop of my blood, extracted as a dark red dense tear from a prick in my right hand middle fingertip.(4). Despite the darkness of the drop, its enlargement on the screen was vanishing pink, with fragmented outskirts indicating, as the biologist explained, weakness of the nervous system cells. Not a word about the pale colour which I thought was the natural one at that scale but that, I had understood later, when the damage was repaired, indicated how debilitated was my system.

Lack of Vitamin C as well as Candidasis in the intestine were detected together with the "hole", which she indicated on the screen with her pen," in the breast area". A remarkable picture not limited to the incriminated part and yet contextualizing it. Further enlargements of the picture and related printouts were made and taken to the next door office for the energy reading section, which was carried out by the biologist's husband.

"Why have you done this to yourself?" was his immediate response to the print outs. This was followed by a verbal picture of my energies detected by handling a special tool. "You are suspended between earth and sky and you can go either way. It is up to you to decide. We can help you only if you choose to come down". Correct. I was not sure I wanted to come down. Did I want to live? Not exactly. Did I want to die? Apparently not.

The diagnosis confirming all Dr. Kingsley's principles based on physiology was very reassuring and confirmed that the thread I had been holding since London was very fine but unbroken. I was indeed affected by an evident lack of Vitamin C, thus by a decreased cellular immunity, which would produce, I was learning, a reduced resistance to fungal infections such as the one I was affected by, Candidasis, produced by Candida, a fungus belonging to our body's flora and member of the yeast family. The bread-less and beer-less diet I was on, was not just a credible abstract dogma, but the perfectly appropriate and convincing creed I continued to practice.

The cure prescribed by the couple was in accordance with the principles discovered in London and it specifically took the form of a discipline mainly consisting in looking after my little girl, myself as a little girl. I was prescribed homework that became my new full time job. Hours were spent in the preparation of a juice obtained by draining a blend of brown rice and kamut that had boiled for almost two hours in a specific number of litres of water. The juice, with a few drops of natural remedies, including lemon extract, added to it, was to be drunk within two days in a specific number of glasses at specific hours. On top of this, aiming to heal the intestine, I prepared all meals as I would have loved to have them prepared for me, with ingredients containing antioxidants in order to boost the immune system and excluding chocolate, meat, milk and cheese.

The entire day was rhythmically articulated by the many dark caramel brown small bottles of assorted shapes, filled with herb extracts and by the various number of drops to be poured out of them into a tablespoon or teaspoon, to be drunk pure or in small cups or glasses of water. This was recommended to be a low PH one, easy to obtain in chemist shops, in glass bottles, that eventually could be delivered at home. Timing and doses were written down in a carefully made schedule, which also included taking a few pills. I stayed mostly at home and, when I needed to move even for a few hours, it was indeed like having to take along a baby, only the pampers and baby carriage were missing.

In addition to making me aware of my bodily needs and of a being embodied, about which I still seemed puzzled, there was a psychological healing involved in all the prescribed procedures. The unwanted child, the one who until youth had always been mothering her mother, was receiving plenty of unusual attention or at least, for the first time she was noticing it. A straightforward explanation could have been that I still needed to be the daughter I had never been in order, eventually, to became a mother. Wasn't I already mother of my projects, helping them to grow with dedication, passion and attention? And yet there was a resistance towards being a mother, a non interest in being one. Nice to be a daughter though, nice to look after myself.

I was aware that the gravity of the disease was in direct ratio to the depth of the problem, therefore that such simplistic explanations were not the primary cause nor the solution; it was still essential to start from the obvious, that I could detect, and progressively leaf through to the core.

Humbled between the fear of dying and the fear of being forced to live, I was aware of having driven myself towards death by being in denial, by ignoring my personal needs for the sake of accomplishing grand ideals advocating for women's needs and rights at birth, promoting worldwide new types of delivery rooms, designing, patenting and producing a pool for comfortable deliveries for mothers and babies and surrendering to the fact of having only a shower for myself, deprived of the pleasure of those baths so vital to my comfort and well being. I had left behind my significant rituals, including music and contemplation, in order to socially fight a de-humanizing routine which most women underwent easily.

Birth, breast. I wasn't a mother nor had I ever desired to become one. I was capable of feminine giving, but having a child would have been the equivalent of the little pool I had designed in relation to the big sea. Motherhood, the feminine and unconditional love were not necessarily related to child and birth, but why was I so focused on the topics and why a cancer so explicitly pointing out a serious conflict in the sexual creative sphere?

Indeed the spontaneous softness of my creative drives had to become hardened to survive. I had to fight professionally in a male world in order to propose a feminine, caring way of designing in an impersonal institutionalized realm, primarily commercial, thus focused on the financial well being for the investors and the powerful rather than the users. Not surprising then that a tough stone had materialized within the softest nourishing organ close to the heart. Was it there to draw the attention to an ignored sacrifice? A warning I believed I was starting to understand.

Was the suffering coming from the heart? Was my giving through work a misplaced love? Did I have the courage to love or was I still expecting somebody to do so with me, possibly out of admiration for my great gestures as a professional child? I was a paradox of contorted femininity aiming to androgynous survival by caring for women in a world of men, refusing to be simply a woman, to accept a codified role, to be in the shadow of a more or less illustrious man, to be the unconditionally loving one. I was the hunting Diana playing and flirting with Apollo and Pan instead. I was Minerva as well, proud of having been born out of Jupiter's head, without the least desire to be Juno, his wife.

Unobtainable, like a deer, watching from far away, higher up in the hills, between bushes and rocks, climbing alone, appearing and disappearing, hunted and not yet aware of her faith. Deep down knowing that a day would come when she would stop, turn her face and look into her hunter's eyes, ready to fall under his arrow and fulfil her destiny by choosing to surrender.

Unable to give a sense to the ordinary, rather running away from it, pick pocketing intellectually, from books, adventures, ideas, stretching my luck, as I had been told just before a train crash I had been involved in, only to survive brilliantly thanks to the angel, the one constantly grabbing me on the verge of falling into the precipice. Thus I used to reassure my mother when concerned about my unconventional life. My 'wagon-lit' was literally there, partially cantilevered and stuck in a precarious balance, with its overweight half over the void and the other half, where my cabin was, suspended above ground where I found myself, in the middle of the night, after having been extracted with my suitcase through the train window.

Unscheduled analytical thinking processes were constantly arising. Was I again stretching my luck then, was there a luck at all to be stretched? Certainly there was an angel.

Meanwhile the time came for the appointment with the channel of my spiritual guide, whom I wanted to hear in order better understand and fully trust my chosen path. "You are carrying the corpses of your lack of compassion." he said. "In wars, even the bodies of the worst enemies are honoured with burial. It has not been so in your life. Your body is disseminated with unearthed rotting corpses waiting for you to bury them. This is what needs to be done. Do this and no trace of disease will be left. Nothing to say to your world when it will address you by stating that you are healed. You would have simply done what needed to be done".

"How can I bury them", I asked, "Whom do I have to bury?" "You will find them anywhere you look in your life and for each of them you will define the appropriate burial." was the answer.

While looking after myself as a child I thus started to face my many selves I had killed as children, youths, adults and other victims of which I have been the murderer. I could detect 57 corpses including other people I metaphorically killed with manifested or un-manifested deliberate action or thought. I hardly remember them, their names drafted in a tiny note book flooded with tears: boys, men, father, mother, behaviours and most importantly the many different forms of myself. Lying abandoned on a rusty earth, dusty, asleep, inert and serene, they had all been taken one by one, revisited and recollected to be laid on a pyre of wood lit beside the ocean, lowered inside a tree trunk, burnt on the shore of a small island, driven to float on a raft towards the horizon, concealed under a blanket of leaves, hidden in a basket of fresh flowers, dissolved as ashes in rivers or lakes, three bodies together buried in the white sand. All fading away in the foggy smoke of my running eyes while I was still not sure whether I wanted to live or not.

Susan had just come from London to help the little girl of me to look after herself: fresh vegetables and fish at the piazza Vittorio market, the delicious black sea bass I devoured and more, possibly anything I could have been eating that day as out of starvation when all of a sudden my little girl, in the midst of that compulsory intake affirmed "yes, I am here, fully on earth". It only occurred to me afterwards that the night before I had dreamt of a new born baby.

I had just received the invitation from Plymouth University to join, like the previous year, a full time teaching week on Humane Architecture at the Schumacher College in Dartington. "Don't go", "you can't", "you shouldn't" were the friendly and supportive voices around me, but I said yes and with all the bottles and remedies complements supplements implements, I went. Corpses were buried and I was getting better and stronger fully dedicated to the discipline of looking rigorously after myself. On a further meeting my spiritual guide had informed me that most of the work I could do alone at that stage was done and nobody but the two of us knew how I was feeling.

It was spring 1998 and, although I was getting better and better, I did not feel any reduction of the lump. It had undergone a change of shape, the nipple was less pulled in, less hidden between the flesh and my energy was positive and light. The biologist and her husband noticed an overall improvement of my blood picture, but no way to make my system assimilate vitamin C, whose intake was always washed out.

My boyfriend, tired of my obsession, tired of having our world revolving around my right breast was showing me brochures on mastectomy, purposely sent to him from England. Such excellent sketches making the intervention simple and normal as it is, as it should be, as it needs to be. Dear Paola from Milan was reminding me of humility, "Now that you have done so much and have been working on compassion, do not forget humility. You are like everybody else, and without pride accept what everybody else does. Go through the operation, remove the lump and solve the problem for good".

After all, according to everybody, I had cancer and even my brother mentioned the disease to the mother of a missed husband of mine, professor and head of one of the oncology departments in Northern Italy, who offered his total help and support in the name of our long and meaningful relationship. I was without medical monitoring and I highly appreciated his kindness.

When I met him at the Institute and showed him the diagnosis, exams and screens and Reports, I explained my focus on boosting the immune system rather than going for chemotherapy. As a consequence he immediately visited my other brother, warning him that I had four months to live. I never understood why not three or five. Certainly my brother became very alarmed.

"Let's go for the mastectomy", I started thinking, "Life has to go on. I have done what I could to heal the cause. Let's remove the lump that is still here". I wasn't ill, for sure, at least not as ill as I had been. I was getting close to the decision mainly to reassure others, to remove their anxiety by undergoing like everybody the sacrifice and relieve myself of you.

I had not brought any nighties nor slippers with me when I had to face the hospitalisation because of the operation and I forced my sister – in - law to supplement my negligence by buying them just before being taken to the hospital by her husband. My younger brother took me there and Andrea came to meet us at the reception almost as if for lunch or dinner or supper, for an aperitif or a cup of tea. I did not have my National Health card either, nor did I remember its number and we called my GP who luckily was in his surgery and by chance answered the phone only to dictate the code to me. It was Wednesday May 13th. My mother's name day and I was there for an operation, booked for the following day.

"There is a nurses strike tomorrow", the receptionist said to Andrea, "we can put her down for Friday". "No, on Friday I am in Sicily for a convention", he replied. "Please put me down for Friday", "No way" said Andrea, "you cannot be alone in the operating theatre. I need to be there". Therefore, unavoidably I was booked for the following Monday.

In preparation for the cuts I would undergo I had started taking marigold pills and had arranged for a Reiki master to come before and after the operation. "Always the same, you have to be different, the treatment is not allowed", Andrea said at first, before softening the reaction, by adding that the therapist would have to come to the ward as a friend of mine and treat me without anybody seeing us.

It was like being in a 3 star hotel with shared rooms and bathrooms. No way to go down to the reception though or to eat in the dining room. Food was announced with the steel noise of shaky trolleys and a vague refectory smell. No nutrition. Very overcooked bleached rice and 'hormonized' boiled chicken corpses were the first day's menu. Tasteless energy-less food, nauseating and revolting because of the careless catering and lifeless service, providing an a-nutritional food, flavour-less and colour less. No minerals left, no vitamins, not to mention antioxidants, a mass of debilitating food and air. How can one be cured here? What a joy was the cooked apple brought in from her home by a nurse, who offered us a cup as her precious gift. Something to look forward to. The only good memory about that place. Simple apples deliciously tasting of apples.

Uncomfortable chairs, pre-second world war style. It was indeed like being in the army, awakened at 5.30, taken temperature, no way to move your pillow to the other side of the bed, simply to be more comfortable while conversing with my next bed neighbour accurately chosen by Andrea as my room mate. Still carrying tubes and bags as a consequence of a surgical intervention to remove cancer from her intestine she was, according to him, the best person for me to share the room with, and indeed she was to the point of the two of us wanting to carry on our conversation by looking at each other while laying or sitting in our beds. Thus I moved my pillow from its orthodox place to opposite end of the bed, where feet were expected to be positioned as I had learned in my visits and research on American hospital design and layouts: reciprocity of two beds positioned opposite each other rather than aligned, created communication and dialogue between people in case they wanted it. Separation and privacy could have been created by a screen or curtain between them.

Heavily reproached by a male nurse, appointed to take my electrocardiogram, I repositioned the pillow where it was supposed to be in order to make him at least not upset. How did I dare to have such a revolutionary initiative interfering with protocol and routine? Wasn't I supposed to be an obedient object parked there while waiting to be saved through surgical mutilation? Wasn't I the patient? Therefore there wasn't any reason for him to be patient with me. I was the one supposed to be a patient patient with him, in obedience even for the Nonsense.

Wednesday and Thursday were lived by feeling like an alien; healthier than everybody else, nurses and doctors included. Feeling perfectly well also when the three heads of departments: the surgeon, the anaesthetist, the plastic surgeon with their charismatic uniforms, like informal archbishops without a tiara, surrounded my bed and started to discuss the cutting of my breast. With a green felt pen the plastic surgeon, designed a sort of eye including the nipple, as the pupil in the Horus Egyptian symbol, missing the elegant tail though. As a designer I suggested modifying the shape of the eye to reduce the cut, whose layout I regret not having taken a picture of out of discretion towards myself.

"Can't you reduce the cut ?" I was asking. "We need to remove as much as possible in order to be on the safe side, since you do not want to undergo chemotherapy. We shall insert a small balloon with a valve that will remain on the skin surface. Slowly we shall inflate the balloon through the valve. Eventually, if no more cancer cells are generated, the balloon will be removed and replaced with a muscle from your body". I did remember Renata, both breasts removed, muscle from her stomach inserted and no muscle in the stomach area to hold it any more, no muscle to lift herself up after having bent over either. Still involved, furthermore, in a court case because her mastectomy was not needed due to the non pathogenic cells, detected from the biopsy report delivered after the operation.

In order for the three of them to be present at the same time on the following Monday, phone calls were made to reschedule my operation to 6.30am. Good. They looked pleased and I imagined I was supposed to be the same having the advantage of being treated in such a privileged way.

As soon as they left I looked at my next bed neighbour. "Are you going to stay?" she asked. "Not sure, at least I'd like to go away for the week end". "Impossible", Andrea said, when I mentioned my desire, "but, if you come back on Sunday afternoon we can arrange for it".

My lady next bed suggested to take all my belonging and place one of her shirts on my side of the cupboard in order not to arouse suspicion and to keep the place booked for me in case I would have decided to go back. Nobody understood that I had taken everything with me, having brought so little in the first place.

I signed and left the hospital with Andrea who dropped me off at the motorway exit where my young brother was supposed to come and collect me. He was supposed to pick me up and take me to his home, 30 kilometres away from the hospital, for the week-end, but I went to the railway station instead and jumped on the first train to Rome, 490 kilometres away, where I could not imagine I would be overwhelmed by the anxieties of the loving ones, all upset by my decision which wasn't yet a decision. I just could not stand the hospitalisation nor was I sure that the cutting would have been the best solution.

Nobody there had a clue nor could I explain what I was going through and those who seemed to have a clue could not support my decision of going ahead in such an unorthodox way. Sergio from Milan was begging me over the phone, that he would take a flight to Rome and take me back to the hospital. My boyfriend was very upset," I don't' love you for your breast, you are not your breast..." and so forth.

Wasn't I the person preaching for freedom of movement in birth places? Wasn't I the one inspired by mammal behaviours in advocating for choice and control at birth? Wasn't the woman symbiotically attuned to her baby, wasn't she supposed, according to my theories deduced from life, to listen to the child and herself, and nobody else, in order to let birth happen? How many times Michel Odent (6) had told me of women hiding behind grand pianos, velvet curtains, tables, sofas and even in bathrooms to handle birth their own way?

I thus locked myself in my bathroom, ignoring phone calls and loving words, sitting on a rather uncomfortable bidet, trying to listen to myself. It was Saturday May 16th, my birthday. When I felt ready and comfortable in my choice I came out of my retreat and faced the first disappointed one. We didn't argue, no point. I was immovable. The decision had been taken. The body was mine.

How to inform the hospital though? And Andrea? I caught him while washing his car in the familiar villa where I was supposed to live had I married him instead of parting. I had to come to terms with the only doctor who would put up with my choices and negotiate with him by adapting to his mindset since he was doing his best to adapt to mine and so I asked him if I could have chemotherapy instead of a mastectomy as a birthday present. "Since you have decided to infer such a big cut on my body because I do not want to go through chemical treatment, I have decided to undergo it first in order to reduce the lump and thus the cut". I was playing for time. I needed to make my decision to sound rational and thus acceptable to his sense of responsibility.

"A wrong decision of yours had killed 'somebody' years ago", I heard him saying "a wrong decision of yours now may kill you" - he said so kindly – "but I cannot but accept it. One request only: you are the one who is going to communicate your decision to the Hospital and to the chief surgeon." From his point of view when I left him years ago I had killed him, and by not going back to the hospital I would have literally killed myself. From my point of view those choices had been my only means to celebrate my life by manifesting dignity.

I breathed out deeply as I still do in describing and remembering. The first part was done. The second would be harder, but the process had started and, by having Andrea as witness, I had entered a path of no return.

I called the Hospital on Sunday afternoon to announce that I would not be returning and that I would personally speak to the professor the following morning.

I did not call him at 6.30, not at 7.00, not at 8.00, nor at 8.30. It was almost 9.00 when I dared. "Yesterday evening, when I heard there was a phone call from the Hospital", he said, "I knew it was about you not coming back. Let me tell you that I felt relieved and I am pleased with your decision. You were not ready for it and would not have forgiven me or yourself for the operation. After chemotherapy the lump will be reduced and intervention will be less invasive. Do start chemotherapy as soon as possible and I shall see you after that."

I was so pleased with his words, his concern, his sensitivity and humanity.

Bibliography

1 – The unbearable image – Raphael Lopez-Pedraza Spring Journal 1996.

2 – Architecture Inside Out – Karen A Frank and Bianca Lepori - Academy Press (March 2000)

3 – O.Carl Simonton, James L.Creighton and Stephanie Mattews Simonton Getting Well Again: A Step-by-step, Self-help Guide to Overcoming Cancer for Patients and Their Families (Pathway) (Paperback – Nov 14, 1986)

4 – Blood smear test. This method is an empirical diagnostic method in medical science that makes possible a found statement on the total condition of the body- Description from: http://www.naturklinik.com/en/clinic/blood-smear-test.php

5 – Selling water by the River: Manual of Zen Training by Jiyu Kennett Vintage February 1974

6 – Michel Odent – Birth Reborn Birth Works (September 1994)

CHAPTER 3

MIND, EMOTIONS AND CANCER: LEARNING FROM NEUROSCIENCE THE BIOCHEMISTRY OF THE UNCONSCIOUS MIND

PARADOXICALLY IT TOOK THE courage and the determination of the Amazon, accustomed to fighting in a male world, to avoid the physical amputation of the right breast by remaining loyal to the feminine as an intuitive way of being. While perpetuating the myth of the *A-matzos*, from the Greek, those without a breast, "female heroic warriors, who were not fearing impediment of whatsoever knight" (1) I was nevertheless concentrated in ignoring diktats, more precisely 'orders imposed by someone in power without popular consent' by doing only what I felt was deeply necessary for myself as a whole being, rather than challenging dogmas as I had been doing prior the diagnosis.

Quickly again back to London, I first went to Bloomsbury to meet the lady doctor known for preventing breast cancer by rebalancing the hormone system and immune systems with natural progesterone, obtained from an exotic plant of the yam family. Chemical progesterone, I was learning, was also derived from a natural element such as pregnant horse urine, information, which confirmed how precious substances were discharged through the golden liquid and also made me realize that, maybe, having continued with the intake of amaroli, I could have even rebalanced my hormone system.

The doctor listened carefully to my story and, of her own initiative, invited me to have another biopsy before starting chemotherapy: "with all you have done you might have transformed the lump", she said, and prescribed natural progesterone (2) to be regularly spread over both my breasts. Distributed as a cream in a white tube, smaller than toothpaste with a very pale blue wisteria writing, it had no pharmaceutical connotation, but rather was very feminine, like a beauty product.

I concluded my trip by going to Ainsworth, the homeopathic pharmacy where, according to doctor Kingsley, one could send her own chemotherapy protocol and receive within two days the homoeopathic remedies that could counteract its damages. Having taken all the information and fax numbers to get on with the necessary procedures, should I choose chemotherapy, I left with all the essential reassuring links.

Back in Italy I was introduced by Andrea to another lady doctor, the head of the department of the day clinic where the chemotherapy sessions would take place. The answer to my request for a second biopsy was negative: "As far as I understand you have not done anything, thus the diagnosis has not changed: since there was cancer there still is cancer. Please do look after yourself: be careful not to get the flu." It was the end of May and she was insisting with me to be mindful about not catching cold. One seldom does in late Spring/ Summer unless lacking vitamin C. She obviously was aware of my deficiency of antioxidants and weak immune system, which favoured cancer growth, but she did not prescribe plenty of Vitamin C instead of or in addition to the warning. "Let's meet and start the therapy in a week's time" was her way of softly inserting another piece on her experimental assembly line.

When I returned she wasn't there, being home with flu, and a young *dottoressa*, a highlighted blond stereotype, was replacing her in order to get me started anyway. Maybe her chief doctor was in the ward and simply passed on the ordinary job of filling in forms with weight, height and extrinsic info prior to formulating the protocol accordingly. The colour of the eyes was not required.

Opposite each other, we sat at a desk just below the air conditioning filter, in which I could observe greasy, dusty grey filaments floating elastically each from its unique suspension spot in the grid just above us. Such a healthy environment! Every now and then one question from her, or from me: "Do you have any suggestion to prevent hair from falling out during the chemo treatment?" "We were using for a while iced rubber hats. Their aim was to freeze the hair bulb while the liquids were injected, but they turned out to cause headaches, and so we are not using them any more". "I understand. "Do you know of any homoeopathic way to solve the problem?" No reply."I see that you have written Tamoxifen. Are you going to prescribe this to me?" "Yes". "I have read that Tamoxifen is an effective hormone therapy against breast cancer but may produce ovarian cancer". "Yes true, but ovarian cancer cases are a small percentage of the total amount of breast cancer cured" "I understand".

Not intending to agree with the 'rigour of the approximation' I was undergoing, I permitted myself to tell the neat and clean young *dottoressa* that her boss, during our previous meeting, had anticipated that she would ask for another biopsy before starting the chemotherapy.

"Let's do it immediately, then". I believe she made a phone call. What I remember is her leading me through corridors to a dark room where another lady biologist with a colleague instantly covered my breast with the cold jelly essential for the x-rays procedure to direct the biopsy.

As soon as the scan of my breast was on the screen, the biologist pronounced loudly a very rude word followed by "Who is your doctor?" "Professor X" was my reply. "There is no cancer lump here, only cysts" and she started removing them by filling three syringes, which I could see were full of the most utterly blessed, blissful liquid.

I could sing I could fly and called my boyfriend in Rome, "Coming back with an empty breast, without the operation. Hallelujah!"

"We need to operate anyway to understand what has happened" was the comment of the biologist a few days later while she was showing me the report of the biopsy ascertaining the presence of cysts and carcinogenic debris. "No way". "Then come back for a check up in 2 months time".

Having gone back I do not remember her second report but I do clearly remember her observation: "If I were you I would get rid of both breasts anyway in order to live for another 5 years". A good enough observation to never go back again. My reply to her, before disappearing for good was "What if a tile falls from a roof and hits me while walking in the street just after the operation?"

If there was a fight going on it had not been against my cancer, but rather in protecting it and myself against orthodox cancer fighters. I was so glad to have listened to myself with the support of my spiritual guide and a few trustworthy unconventional professionals authors and friends. The life scholars, the searchers, the intelligent, the creative ones, the ones impossible to pin down to official notions, the outsiders, ancient souls with a deep connection to a clear source, the ones moving with confident grace on a path of uncertainty based on taking responsible risks, the ones accepting individuality, without fearing death, acknowledging it instead as part of living, the ones dreading more than disease the surrender to the ignorance of an allopathic approach to health aimed at dis-empowering people by taking away their individual control.

Likewise I needed to protect myself from other agents of the Health field. The producers of a birthing pool I had designed patented and co-produced were attacking me in my work territory. My shared investment in the newly produced innovative product was evolving into a few sales obtained exclusively through my promotions but absolutely no profit was shared with me by the producer who was, as a matter of fact, denying any right I had by the contract he was breaching, as if there wasn't one.

Equally in the Health sector, of the two prototypes for birth and community centres I had promoted and made a preliminary innovative design for in Tuscany, one had been commissioned, for the working drawings part, to a colleague with a curriculum in cemeteries rather than in birthplaces. Despite what could have seemed an evolved choice, implying the analogy between death and birth as rites of passage, there was not such a spiritual and enlightened motivation in the appointment. The colleague had won the competition by illegally reducing to zero his fees for professional expenses thus overcoming by 0.027 my credits based on my exclusive skill on the topic.

In the meantime, the administration of the same hospital in Florence was trying to skip paying my fee for the preliminary design, upon which the competition had been based. I was forced to have a solicitor involved and take the Careggi Hospital to court, immediately coming to an agreement simply because of the administrator's fear of being blackmailed: a public institution cannot put up for tender a project that is not his own because it has not been paid. With all my thanks to the potential scandal that came to my aid, for the first and last time, I got quickly and straightforwardly hold of what was mine.

Meantime the United Hospital of Brescia, where I had been appointed to upgrade 10.000 sqm of the maternity department, to include the neonatal ward, ended up sending, by ordinary mail and against our written agreement, the balance check of 42 million lira, equivalent to approximately 30.000 dollars. The envelope, not registered, went lost, without my knowing whether it had ever been sent while the hospital refused to wire the amount to my bank account as had been agreed in the contract. To do so, after a first approved payment, another board meeting was needed and, in the meantime the check might have reached my address. As always happens in our profession, most of that money had been used to pay other people collaborating on the task. This to be added, in my case, to the cost of the eccentric health treatments that were entirely paid for by myself.

I was full of rage bouncing against all those rubber walls. It took a few months to sort out the purposely set up negligence of Brescia hospital while the relationship deteriorated and while the administration acquired the strategic layout of my plans. Once again in my career, other colleagues, without knowledge of the topic, were appointed; with the consequence of de-naturalizing the project. Nevertheless they, rather than I, took the credit for the results, which were deprived of their contents during the process.

The skill, care and cure given to my creations were regularly exploited and stolen and I was most often financially abused. The experience with birth places, as with my disease, brought me to realize how unhealthy can be a Healthcare System that is uniquely a business, refusing any innovation that reduces medicalization and that is based on, as in the case of the Careggi Hospital, in Florence, favouring of political liaisons.

Since the health care field is characterized by products that are expensive because of the degree of safety and technology performed as well as expected from them, the producer of the pool I had patented and co-produced as well as carefully and knowledgeably designed in order to be ergonomically functional and beautiful, took over by adding, without my consent, unneeded technology to the fibre glass shell. As a consequence, thanks to his technological know-how, which was unnecessary and out of my control, it raised the selling price to an outrageous amount with the result that only a few pools were sold and I lost both professional credibility and financial reward.

Not only did my birthing pool no longer appear coherent with my preaching, its natural calmness and harmony, were destroyed by the engine noise of unnecessary water jets and other rough last minute added details. I also had to put up with being the inventor of the gigantic phallic box. This out- of -proportion command board, two meters tall, sixty centimetres wide and thirty deep, was meant to house three or four switches and had been produced from an old cast that was lying around in the factory, having been used, years before,

BIANCA LEPORI

to manufacture a command board commissioned for the Army. Not difficult to acknowledge, from the literal combination of a carefully and purposely uterus shaped pool and an anonymous penis-moulded absurdity, how once again men were coming in and abusing a female field with their phallic ignorant and greedy arrogance, which deprived the result of a creation, filtered by tens of mindful meetings with midwives, obstetricians and pregnant women.

I had come out of a health tunnel, only to find myself in a loathsome health care one. After only a few months from the escaped mastectomy and chemotherapy, a lump in my breast materialized again and pain started to trouble my right armpit. Soon I began to follow very fast cells running down like mercury drops along my arm, just above the wrist. No, not again. I was too busy surviving professionally and financially. I did not have the time to start again with the boosting procedures. Thus I decided to give in to like-minded doctors without realizing how that would mean loosing even further control.

I was in a circuit of ecologists and friends who suggested I make an appointment with the most reliable holistic doctor in Rome, well known for his ortomolecular medicine and mindful of physiological balance and diet. He was practising Hulda Clark Zapping and prescribing the Di Bella cure, which was very popular those days, thanks to recurrent television debates between the head of the most modern and famous oncology hospital in Milan and the elderly doctor who had formulated the multi-therapy named after him. Applied privately outside the national healthcare system, his medical approach to cancer was based on a blend called *Somatostadine*, on an antioxidant syrup and, essentially, on the one-to-one relationship with him. It was the semi-orthodox therapy closest to my search and understanding, potentially capable of having an effective impact on the ongoing inability of my system to absorb Vitamin C.

I would have liked to meet Dr. Di Bella and have the therapy tailored to me by him, but the waiting list was too long and so I decided to go for the sensitive holistic Roman doctor who could immediately prescribe that therapy to me. Not only did I know him, but I had listened to his brilliant lectures, read his books and had even spoken at the same conference once. During the initial visit he immediately detected a violence I had undergone as a child by my father, an observation rather shocking to me, until of course I remembered the wound. Our dogs, the two German shepherds I had grown up with in the woods, were killed, I always believed, when we moved from the mountains to the lake. Because of the mysterious way of taking them away from us, I imagined he had them killed, in that village at the end of that straight road intersecting the wide bend on the Stelvio state road. There, where a few years later he had a serious car accident which I avoided by chance, insisting to remain with my grandparents instead of leaving them and accompanying him and my little brother to collect my mother. I never asked about the dogs, maybe they have been kept happily alive, but the car accident at that precise point had since been a secret motive of uneasiness and pain. After all I had grown up with these dogs, accustomed to their presence, loyalty and intelligence and I forever felt the injustice of the loss.

Never asked, as I didn't when afterwards I fell so much in love with that grey squirrel which I saw for the first time on a walk through the hazelnut trees. I felt so compelled that I wanted my father to buy one for me, but I did not make any request. Was that for the sake of the squirrel I so strongly felt should not to be deprived of its freedom or was it my fear of eventually being deprived of it as well? A formula was coming to light almost as an instruction given to myself by myself about avoiding what could make me happy in order not to suffer for its unavoidable loss.

The doctor prescribed as expected the "Di Bella treatment" together with other remedies that would integrate it. Being a friend he kindly waived his consultancy fee and pointed out that the remedies and chemicals had to be bought in two different Chemistry shops: most of them could be found just outside the Vatican, while the chief ingredients of the Di Bella cure, which were *Somatostadine* and the antioxidant syrup, could be bought at the Chemist under the Piazza della Repubblica arcade.

I went first towards the Vatican area where the chemist knew what I was after and asked if I was aware that I could buy *Somatostadine* at a controlled price. Nobody had told me this, but I was feeling quite comfortable since the addresses of both chemistry shops had been given to me by a doctor friend.

The second prescription for the second chemist indicated 4 doses of *Somatostadine* I needed to start buying in order to have two injections a week during the upcoming fortnight. I clearly remember the setting and the play. "Five hundred lira" said the second chemist while coming back triumphantly to the desk holding, together with the prescription, one small box. "We have only one dose. Come back next week with one million and half for the other three". "I want to heal, not to get sick even further", I replied.

Smiling, he looked at me with an arrogantly paternalistic face commenting: "This product is fantastic but expensive. It requires a wallet like this" – and parted his hands ten centimetres while keeping them parallel - "People sell their homes in order to afford it." And he was probably going to buy them thanks to it.

I left the box on the desk and saved the five hundred, approximately equivalent to 350 dollars. It was evening I remember, and rather dark. I needed to get on with finding the chemist shop that was selling *Somatostadine* at a controlled price. Maybe with one million lira I could get the first four dosages.

There was an association named after Di Bella in Rome and I had had the opportunity to be introduced to it by two of its members, whom I did not hesitate to call on the following morning to discover that there were three cities in Italy where one could find what I was looking for; one of them was Rome, piazza Bologna where I went with my prescription asking to start with the first box only. The price was announced to be fifty three thousand lira, one tenth of the previous day's asking price, which was aligned with corporate standards and obviously included my fee to my doctor friend.

Somatostadine needed to be injected with a temporized syringe, and therefore I had to buy one. The chemist of piazza Bologna gently came back from the rear of his shop with another box, an oblong one, like the one of fountain pens. "Seven hundred fifty thousand lira"."Sorry? Is there a way of sharing one with another person? After all we need it only once or twice a week". He almost laughed at me.

I left with the *Somatostadine* but without the temporized syringe, which, after a few phone calls, I discovered could be bought in Perugia at less than half the price: 350.000 lira approximately. I thus went to Perugia to buy one and came back to Rome with two for free, donated by G who had been experimenting with everything and was struggling in the very late stages.

What was very good of the Di Bella's protocol was the antioxidant syrup, different from one Chemist Shop to another I came to realize. I had learned where to find the best one, dense purple red, almost like a flavored nourishing blood. Di Bella's multi-therapy consisted of a five-substance therapy made with two hormones: *Somatostadine* and melatonin, retinoids, vitamins and small doses of some chemotherapeutic agents. All these were mixed in the *Somatostadine* blend that was a nightmare if you wanted to inject it on your own. At least it was for me, absolutely unfit to face let alone personally deal with any medical technicality.

Once filled with the liquid, the syringe was inserted in the temporizer where a time was established for the liquid to pour out and enter your system in a monitored time of approximately six or eight hours, corresponding roughly to an average sleeping time. The needle, with a plastic butterfly or dragon-fly, that I remember as being yellow, was inserted into the belly just below the navel and one was supposed to sleep in a position that would not allow the needle to fall off the skin. Band-aids were contributing to the task. After five injections I gave up, perceiving the therapy as absolutely useless, except for the syrup that I carried on buying. More tailored on the 500.000 lira than on myself, the therapy I had been prescribed wasn't the one I was aiming for.

Professor Luigi di Bella, an eighty-five-year old physiologist, had been carrying out pharmacological research independently from the Ministry of Health. I remember his interviews full of respect for the people who were crowding into his own house in Modena where he personally adapted his protocol individually to each person, resulting in the one- to- one relationship; the secret of his success. Not surprising that, when an experiment with his protocol had finally been introduced in a few hospitals, it proved not to be effective. It has been commented that, during the trial, instructions had not been followed in the preparation of the components and, as for the ingredients, not even the doses administered were correct. Furthermore it has been reported that the protocol had been applied to people in the 3rd stage of disease who had already undergone chemotherapy, which, according to doctor Di Bella, had a harmful effect on patients.

He ended up being criminalized despite his knowledge and the several people healed by his method. It was very sad to be a spectator to the fight he did not want, and the defensive position taken by the Institutions and the scientific establishment who could not accept such an alternative based on physiology and individual passion. An alternative of uniqueness and criticism, that was too weak compared with the one of institutionalized and officially authorized corporate *mafia*.

He was loosing control, I was loosing control and yet there was nothing more I could do. Biologist and shaman, in the reading of my blood cells, were observing that I was still not assimilating vitamin C and thus the only action required seemed a trip to England again, this time to meet with Dr. Kingsley. I had learned a lot from him about antioxidants, diets and homoeopathic remedies. He was the one who could reverse the process of MS and cancer through vitamin C injections.

I made an appointment and flew to London once again. Maria Claudia drove me to his surgery, which had a very green and domestic atmosphere. He analysed the lump that in the meanwhile had started developing again and put me on two intravenous drips daily, one of 13 grams of vitamin C and one of Oxygen Peroxide, plus one injection a day of oleander extract, which directly addressed the cancer cells due to the poisoning powers of the plant. I left his surgery with lots of bottles, some three thousand pounds lighter, with Maria Claudia thinking the price was immoral.

Aiming to sort out my problem with vitamin C I thought that its elimination was indeed worth the cost of two chemotherapy treatments, which I knew would have been approximately as expensive. The only difference was these seemed cheap because they were offered free to the consumer, at least in Italy. Almost a gift.

I was obsessed with my inability to absorb vitamin C and convinced that the strong intake would force my system to accept it. Furthermore, the oxygen peroxide would have contributed to destroying cancer cells because of their aero phobia. Pancreatic enzymes were also prescribed since it was believed they could attack and liquefy tumours. My remedies would last a month.

Back in Italy I realized that I needed a nurse twice a day: one for the vitamin C drip in the morning, the other for the Oxygen Peroxide one in the afternoon.

100.000 lira a day had already been spent for the two remedies and I was spending the same amount a day for nurses. Cotton wool sometimes was included in the price, though.

I asked my GP if there could be any way around this and he arranged for a day clinic intravenous Vitamin C drip once a day for one week. Oxygen Peroxide being considered only for external use, there was no way to have a drip of that as well. At the end of the week I was sent to the oncology department where another doctor looked so terrified at my breast that I had to beg him not to be afraid. "You need to have an operation". "I am not going to". "As you like, but you have never seen me and I have never seen you. Understood? You have never seen me".

I did not have, in the cancer field, the instruments or the lexicon I had built up for birth places, nor the sounded critique that had allowed me to de-construct and reconstruct them. Being an intellectual, involved in the new learning alternative to mainstream medicine, I could only detach myself from orthodox protocols, whose male culture was reducing care, investigation in human nature and wholeness, to a lace-making activity of some gentle and useless person. A servant in fact.

Doctors are not intellectuals, often not brilliant scientists either. This sentence came to me from the last revelation I had been given, once more, by Veronica. It was from Candace Perth's book *Molecules of emotion – Why you feel the way you feel. (4)* She, the author, as Deepack Chopra foresaw in the introduction to the book, was the first *Western scientist who had done the work of explaining the unity of matter and spirit, body and soul (5).*

It was clear I was moving within such a revolution; perceived and recognised. Only needed to trust it and grasp its scientific evidence. In her book Dr. Pert was very personal, wanting to abolish *the imaginary wall that separates scientists from lay persons.*

There she was, manifesting what I had always felt the need for after reading the article "Out of the academy into the street" by the American author, feminist and social activist, Bell Hooks (6). The longing of these two authors to break the wall of the aristocratic citadel of scientific knowledge and move into personal experience, was also mine. I could clearly see myself standing in the pivotal position similar to the one Candace Perth was in, while defining the new approach to birth and birth places, there at the centre between the right and the left brain functions, in a place of knowledge and synthesis. I had been illustrating them in diagrams to explain the necessary coming together of the opposites of home and the traditional medical hospital birthing rooms, in the place where safety would come from knowing, understanding and listening to the wholeness of an emotionally alive person.

Professionally I had stepped over from architecture to health care by advocating for a natural event such as birth, expressing health and the miracle of nature that would require, environments not exclusively medical in at least 80% of cases. Personally, with cancer, a terrifyingly heavy pathology, I had only followed what seemed the best path for my nature without ever allowing the medical sector to sneak in with a say that could objectively make sense. I was basically searching, hardly finding ways appropriate to my nature, something that could not yet be theorised.

Up until then, my approach to cancer had been unscientific, nothing proven, no similar cases to refer to, a *sui generis* experience that seemed to have developed step by step along a path made of meetings, scattered information, circumstances, coincidences, articles, tapes, people, friends. A personal experience based on intuition, the ancient Egyptian *intelligence du coeur (7)* making a discrimination of what to follow from what not to.

As one doctor said, I had officially simply been an amateur treating myself with Lourdes water. How could one argue with such authority? Daring to break the dogma would have been a childish more than heretical response. Heretical as had been my reply to the priest who reminded me not to look so straight in his eyes because he was a man of God. Did he agree with my comment about myself also being a woman of God?

Candace Pert had the knowledge the intuition and the language. She was and is a pharmacologist and neuroscientist, interested in the crossing over between psychology and physiology; putting together behaviour and chemistry biology. Despite her articulate knowledge she, who could have been eating, as it is said in Italy, over the heads of all doctors I had met until then, she had been teased and laughed at. She had been robbed of her pioneering ideas by colleagues and University professors who had been presenting her papers without mentioning her name on topics she had co-discovered, and using her findings to win prizes instead of her. She suffered, but succeeded in proving the ownership of her discoveries which she so generously gave to *the world*.

There was *"sexism in science"*, she admitted: according to her, Rosalind Franklin, the English pioneer molecular biologist, who was responsible for much of the research and discovery work that led to the understanding of the structure of DNA, *had been dribbled by Linus Pauling.* As a consequence of *the humiliation she suffered at the hands of those "old boys"* to include other colleagues - *her disease had been exacerbated and the failure to express her anger contributed to and possibly caused her death (8)* by ovarian cancer when she was 38.

Was that so stressful and frustrating professional path of mine creating a similar pattern in my system? Emotions, according to Dr Perth had some kind of influence on disease and she had been stubbornly concentrated on proving it.

My eyes were widely open to breath in, digest, metabolize what was clear and yet still so difficult to explain. The thrilling information was about the existence in the body of messenger molecules that were, as she detected in her laboratory, distributing information throughout the organism. As information agents, these molecules, called neuropeptides, were found not only in the cortex, seat of the conscious mind, but also in the emotional brain as well and were distributed throughout the entire nervous system. C*ommunication* therefore *was taking place, not just within the brain but within the rest of the body as well.* (9)

The discovery that indeed peptides were circulating through the body brought Dr Pert to see in the brain the conscious mind, and in the body the unconscious one. *There was then a mind in the body,* she wrote and I took note of it, *a filtering storing learning remembering repressing one. Memories are stored not only in the brain but in a psychosomatic network extending into the body, particularly in the ubiquitous receptors between nerves and bundles of cell bodies called ganglia, which are distributed not just in and near the spinal cord, but all the way out along pathways to internal organs and the very surface of our skin. The decision about what becomes a thought rising to consciousness and what remains an undigested thought pattern buried at a deeper level in the body is mediated by the receptors. I'd say that the fact that memory is encoded or stored at the receptor level means that memory processes are emotion-driven and unconscious.(10)*

According to her, *repressed traumas caused by overwhelming emotion can be stored in a body part, thereafter affecting our ability to feel that part or even move it.(11)* The good news was that there were *infinite pathways for the conscious mind to access the unconscious mind (12)* and I was becoming very intrigued by this possibility.

Bibliography

1 – Publio Virgilio Marone, Eneide, book I.810-814
2 – Natural progesterone: http://www.icnr.com/NaturalProgesterone/NaturalProgesterone.html
3 – Luigi Di Bella: http://www.metododibella.org/en/mdb/home.do
4 – Candace Perth Molecules of emotion The science behind Mind-Body Medicine Simon & Schuster; first edition September 1997
5 – Depack Chopra introduction to Candace Perth Molecules of emotion The science behind Mind-Body Medicine Simon & Schuster; first edition September 1997
6 – Bell Hooks http://www.education.miami.edu/ep/contemporaryed/bell_hooks/bell_hooks.html
7 – Intelligence of the heart Isha Shwaller de Lubicz. Her Back – Egyptian Initiate Hodder and Stoughton; 1St Edition edition (January 1, 1967)
8 – Candace Perth ibidem
9 – Ibidem
10 – Ibidem
11 – Ibidem
12 – Ibidem

CHAPTER 4

VITAMIN C INJECTIONS AND AURIC HEALING: EXPERIMENTING WITH THE REATIONSHIP BETWEEN PHYSICAL AND ENERGETIC BODIES

T HE VITAMIN C AND the oxygen peroxide bottles progressively decreased and after a month I was ready to meet Dr. Kingsley again for a check-up that confirmed the need to continue with the intravenous injections. Since my left arm's veins, damaged by too many perforations, could no longer cope with the therapy and my finances could not continue to bear the cost of nurses, a Hickman line was suggested. This would allow the two chemicals to enter the body through a soft plastic tube inserted into one of the main blood vessels; the superior vena cava. Fixed in such a way to be kept in place for an extended period of time, the device would save me from having further needle pricks and would make me, furthermore, independent from daily nurses. The Hickman line needed to be surgically placed and we called Andrea who agreed for me to have it inserted in his department where a young doctor would be appointed to do so as soon as I returned to Italy.

As explained in advance, local anaesthesia was applied for the small incision to be made in order for the catheter to be introduced and clamped to the skin next to my collar bone, on the left side of my neck. Sealed with a little pale blue plastic butterfly, it ended up sticking out from my décolleté like a pop art broche in need of being protected with colourful scarves.

Blood-phobic as I had always been, I needed to understand and practice the procedure of inserting both the vitamin C and oxygen peroxide, taking care not to let air enter the silicone tube, which, after each injection, needed to be flushed with heparin in order to prevent blood, mine, from clotting. Because of infection that could also be produced by the catheter, attention was paid to the space and worktop were feeding bottles, needles and cotton wool were laying and handled.

I soon learned to carry out the ritual on my own, no longer being afraid of my own blood and became rather comfortable with the practice. I methodically carried on with this until the night in which the Hickman line ended up being obstructed and taken with the body to which it was clamped to the closest emergency room, where it was removed. Only later did I realize that the outpouring side of the inserted catheter was to be positioned at the junction of the superior vena cava and the right atrium of the heart and how, in that point was located the outpouring side of mine too. Despite all the work and the research to become aware of the disease, I was still rather unconscientious, as if aware that the disease was in my body, without the body concerning me.

Blood's drop on the screen at the biologist's studio was bold, strong, dark coloured and alive. The massive intravenous injections had persuaded my system to surrender: "we shall not lack vitamin C any longer", seemed to be the reply of the healthy, vigorous, handsome cells, so unlike the disembodied ones that had appeared on the screen on my first visit. Nevertheless the lump was there again, very stone like, rough under the skin, and tiny arrows were again shooting down from my right arm pit.

Having encountered and been influenced by Candace Perth's vivid description of the relationship between emotion and disease, I could not but see my cancer as a mind body issue and I started to feel rather powerless in the quest ahead to heal both body and mind of it.

Time was passing and Dr. Kingsley, in order to terminate the physical struggle, had mentioned a technique he was exploring in Germany, which consisted of reducing the lump with cold therapy. Its cost was one million a day, equivalent to two somatostadine injections at the standard price.

Now that the immune system seemed to have recovered thanks to the vitamin C, such a high cost could have been justified in order to dissolve the mass once and for all. Despite my curiosity about the conscious/unconscious mind connection I needed to get on with my life, and, having done so much in trying to understand it, I felt the time had come to be helped in quickly getting rid of the carcinogenic mass.

The one million a day fee was inclusive of treatment and full board in the clinic. I wasn't sure whether 10 or 20 days would be needed. My younger brother was willing to offer the money for it and so I contacted the clinic to send me all the necessary information and price schedule. It was the end of summer 1998.

While in the process of booking a room in Germany, I received a phone call from Giulia, a client and friend, owner of the small community "The Angels", from which I had been given the title of 'Architect of the Angels', having designed its refurbishment. Surprised about my health struggle, of which she knew nothing, she exclaimed "I have just heard of a lady in Umbria." and added. "She reads auras and I have been told that she is specifically a cancer healer. I have a meeting booked with her on Tuesday. I can call her and ask to swap my appointment with you".

Instead of changing her date, the healer suggested to Giulia that I could call her on that same evening and she gave me an appointment for the following day, Monday, in a small town, approximately one hour train ride from Rome.

My attitude of reading and accepting signs had just then been stigmatized in the motto that Dr. Perth inherited from the head of her department and that, I in turn, had pencilled in my diary: *Do not accept the conventional wisdom. Do not accept the idea that something can't be accomplished because the scientific literature says it can't. Trust your instincts. Allow yourself a wide latitude in your speculations. Don't depend on the literature – it could be right or it could be completely wrong. Spread all hunches out before you, and go with the ones that you think are most probable. Select the one that you can test easily and quickly. (1)*

I only remember that, after a short conversation, the healer asked me to stand in front of a white partition while facing her. "Some people, she said, bear weights on their shoulders. You are bearing walls".

Her other words have faded away. I only vividly recall her asking me to lie down on a massage bed and, while standing on my left side, she directed her hands first above my forehead, then above my chest and solar plexus. Having then positioned herself on the right hand side of my body, she placed her hands a few centimetres above my right breast. When she removed them I felt the roots of my tumour going away as well, as if she had eradicated the disease from my flesh, as she might have done with a tiny plant and its surrendering loose roots.

I remained where I was, still lying down while she left the room. I did feel it. Very delicately and yet powerfully something big had happened.

What precisely I did not know. Not a single word from her.

Once back in the room again, calmly and quietly, she came towards the massage bed and, knowing perfectly what had happened, and looking into my eyes she whispered "Maybe, instead of going to Germany, you come here".

In pure trust I surrendered to her way of healing that, as I immediately perceived, was to cure the physical by intervening on the invisible.

Having experienced the extraction-uprooting of an ethereal form, almost the essence of the disease, I felt that, with this healer, the lump would dissolve again by having my terrain purified of deeper causes that I could not get to on my own. Indeed a step beyond all the work I had done while burying the corpses of my past and the innumerable complementary techniques I had adopted. If these all, thanks to the conscious work, which was the most I could do on my own, had melted the mass in the first phase, only a priestess, gifted with a view going far beyond my own into the human energy field, could have identified and dissolved deeper wounds and ancestral pains.

At the beginning the treatments had a very intensive schedule: two or three treatments a day, two or three times a week. I had to book a hotel in town to have a rest in between therapies. She was digging out pain from the heart, anger and resentments; clearing out one after the other all the negative emotions that I was going to manifest to the poor man waiting for me at home, regardless of his behaviour. By picking on a word or a gesture I was immediately vomiting out, for the first and last time in my life, all possible negativities and nastiness.

It might be an over simplification to reduce the effects of the therapy to these behaviours. It wasn't clear what exactly was happening. My feeling was that of becoming every day more light, clean and clear, as if slowly coming out of a foggy cloud. I discovered that my healer had been trained by Barbara Brennan (2), the author of "Hands of Light" and it was indeed with her hands of light that she was rebalancing my aura by re-attuning all the energy bodies surrounding my physical one. She did not say or explain anything about her work, but posters in her studio showed the egg shaped diagram of the bodies of light she was working on. They were extending beyond the physical body and contained it, like a set of seven matrioskas dolls contains the seed.

The seven energy bodies were shown as layers of light encapsulating the physical body, each with a specific thickness and colour. What fascinated, and totally convinced me, was the concept of a disease starting outside the physical body in one of the invisible layers surrounding it and moving down or inwards through the lower or innermost bodies, getting closer to the physical one and eventually entering it. Such was the path from dis-easiness to disease. This was the evidence of how the invisible, unbearable image eventually becomes visible. The mechanics, explained in esoteric terms, were mind blowing. It was thrilling, exciting, enough to be joyously happy just to know this method, for how much sense it made and for the reassuring calmness it was creating.

Yes. It made sense. I had found it. No accident, only a marvellous design of causes and effects, a perfectly set up system leading to awareness, responsibility, consciousness. The cause- effect system was perfectly designed and I was safe, so incredibly safe in the womb of a universal knowledge.

Barbara Brennan indeed was a healer, but also a spiritual leader, holding a Doctorate of Philosophy, one of Theology, a Master's Degree in Atmospheric Physics, a B.S. in Physics. She had been working at NASA and was a pioneer and innovator in the field of energy consciousness. All this was perfect for me, since consciousness was indeed my obsession.

It was mind blowing to imagine these layers surrounding my physical body and to have somebody, in unpretentious silence, not only see but work on them, detecting traces that had entered or would have entered the physical to harm me in the flesh once again. My healer only told me that cancer patients have a brown patch outside the body next to the organ in which it has or is going to manifest. According to her, by working on the external bodies the brown mass dissolves and cancer would disappear or not appear in the physical body. It was so wonderful and such a relief to know that the cleansing of the aura would prevent physical disease as well. Her ability to read my other bodies, that I could not see, was quite staggering.

What could she see, how could she see? She was scientifically operating on my energy field, on my outer invisible shells and it was working. It was not only a gift but a lesson since I was healed by somebody, uneasy with words, a doer rather than a talker or a theorizer, as I was inclined to be.

Being scanned by her was much more intimate than going through an x-ray machine. No contrast liquids were needed either. She could see the condition of my physical organs through the reading of their colours in my outer bodies : from the one of my solar plexus she could, for instance, detect the type of relationship I had had in between our meetings. How much she saw and never revealed, I shall never know. From a certain point onwards, while doing her treatments, she placed a pink quartz over my heart, to infuse it with the rose light of love. Indeed my heart was opening immensely. Despite her silence, and thanks to it, I came to realize that I was experiencing Energy Medicine and undergoing Auric Healing. Of this, at least, I needed to be aware. The tumor melted away for the second time, its causes having been eradicated. She did it for me and I was immensely grateful.

By the end of the year, it was 1998, I was totally cleared and my hair from being red had become short and white, with only a few leftover red stripes. I changed gear and moved on, running my small practice full speed, with the help of excellent collaborators, carrying on with the working drawings for the community centre maternity prototype I had been appointed to design. Christmas and New Year's Eve were spent at the office with Maria Claudia and her partner, both having come from London to help me again, this time to get on with practical life "adrenalinically" and meet with me a professional dead line.

Not a penny had been received for the sale of the co-produced as well as designed and patented birthing pools. I had been asking the engineer, their producer and distributor, to at least give me my share as a monthly salary that could have helped me to integrate part of the loss of my health costs. He had been informed of my health condition but, probably since I was not dramatically into traditional therapies, he could not believe it and ignored both my condition and requests.

The solicitor who had brilliantly won the court case against the Careggi Hospital in Florence, was more than happy to set up another court case, against the pool producing company to which only the fair reimbursement was demanded. As a reaction, the company asked us 10 times as much for damages, motivated by a series of lies that I could and did dismantle one after the other.

By June, 1999 I was feeling healed, only somewhat fat and unfit, just in time to start a new relationship with a super-fit brilliant and dynamic colleague.

Bibliography

1 – Candace Perth Molecules of emotion The science behind Mind-Body Medicine Simon & Schuster; first edition September 1997
2 – Barbara Brennan and Jos. A. Smith Hands of light: A Guide to Healing the Human Energy Field Bentam May 1, 1988

CHAPTER 5

REMISSION AND BACK AGAIN: LEARNING FROM FINANCES AND FAILING AS UTOPIAN ENTREPRENEUR

DIFFERENT FROM CURING, HEALING is concerned with rebalancing the luminous nature of beings rather than blindly handling physical manifestations of esoteric causes. I could have jumped off my professional track and followed the new avenue of my recent experience of having regained health in such a logical way.

This would have implied starting from scratch, from the enormous breakthrough of a personal experience that had made me stronger. *Blanche de Force* (1), the name of the famous Poulenc opera protagonist was recurrently coming to my mind and I often referred to it almost like a mantra.

Despite the strength, or because of it, or even because of a disguised weakness, I preferred to keep the experience in the background as an awareness and make what I thought would be a professional step forward by better structuring what was objectively recognized as my know-how.

Something was changing in the birth place scenario. The market seemed to be ripening slightly and, with two obstetricians, I started to bring forward the entire set of furniture for the new model of a delivery room, I had previously sketched and designed and whose production, hopefully, was going to be carried out by an Italian entrepreneur. From the previous years' experience I had grasped the importance of interdisciplinary work and learned the process of bringing ideas into reality as well as acknowledging the slow pace of such an enterprise. It was all very exciting and I could not but decide to carry on working in the maternity field in a creative and more socially responsive way, by contributing to the radical change that I knew was needed in a field I held so much data about, shared with brilliant like-minded people.

I intended to bring all this forward. My curricula, both the professional practice and the health history ones, were concerned with how medicine and architecture are 'non-scientific' when in denial of the holistic. Energy and energy fields had also become paramount in my mind and intentions. Energy was breaking boundaries between professions and categories allowing to be envisaged a cultural revolution of interconnectedness and love for one-another independent of personal relationships.

Interwoven and interdependent, everything was connected to everything.

With the intention of standing out and advocating for these principles, I felt I was equipped with the perfect background to bring forward what was truly interesting and motivating to me: a way of making architecture that would produce awareness, well being and social involvement. In other words an architecture that could be a way of unveiling, deconstructing, naming and reconstructing that which existed, with people rather then only profit in mind.

I had always found that the label 'architect' did not correctly represent my way of practising. I had also felt that the way architecture was thought of and generally practised did not satisfy my social, psychological and environmental beliefs. The focus of architecture was, in schools, mainly on arbitrary aesthetics, whereas in practice, it was definitely on economics. Thus with the chance for us to be professionally successful by offering and adapting our creativity to speculative powers rather than lingering in a niche, like the one I was in, where we would strive to challenge the *status quo*. I considered architecture as a container of ways of being; thus interpreting my professional role as the one of facilitator of these ways. The issue for me was not so much architecture, but rather to be dynamically involved in an ever-changing world, quite the opposite of the frozen built shapes, extraordinary as they could be, rigorous convent walls within which one could be buried alive in a routine of repetitive rituals.

Thanks to the individual path chosen in facing cancer, I had become more aware of the need to promote a way of practising that, likewise, could be supportive of, rather than contrasting, people's nature. I was feeling the urge for an evolution that would break the pattern of casualness, empowering for the few and so dis-empowering for almost everybody else. I was fully dedicated to my profession, believing and longing to contribute to a concept of design that, rather than being a means of giving packaged commercial answers only, could be a way of asking questions and challenging the existing as well. Acting upon environmentally frozen patterns that 'sclerotize' brains and human behaviours had become my conscious mission.

Obviously mine was not one supported by the 'main stream' ways of practice and, having realized that it was the only way for me to actively give and share my beliefs, I had to find a means to move from my individual mode of practising to an officially established one that I would like to contribute to promoting worldwide.

My task was ambitious. Were there MA courses that could help me to operate effectively in such domains? In other words, was there a place, an organisation where I could get the skill to further my goal, a label that would give me the authority to operate?

"Here is your School", a friend pointed out. I had never heard of the School for Social Entrepreneurs (2) in London before. I looked at the program, discovering that I had all the qualities implied: being a visionary almost possessed by my ideas, ambitious, persistently committing my life to changing the direction of my field, offering new ideas for wide-scale change, initiator and promoter of social change. Furthermore I realised that my way of conceiving my practice was precisely the one of a social entrepreneur, interested in topics pertaining to the public sector, in which it could not invest, while the private sector would not find enough return to financially commit.

The course would last one year and consist of classes finalized to help students to consolidate their own projects by setting up their own organisation. I applied to the School and was accepted. The project I proposed sounded like:'Society for women centred childbirth' its mission being the one of encouraging and facilitating a worldwide transformation of the current practice of child delivery. The Society would have my healing experience as anonymous and personal background and be the continuation of my professional practice over the last 12 years. Its purpose would be that of effectively promoting a global transformation in the field, like Margaret Sanger (3) or Maria Montessori (4) successfully did with the movement for family planning and the approach to child education respectively.

Through a holistic approach to childbirth, by focusing on woman and child as whole human beings, the project would aspire toward reintegrating into the birth experience and consequently into birth places, the values dismissed by contemporary 'one-sided' medicalization.

Despite the drive to change, as architect I could not nevertheless act toward changing the status quo of birth places as I individually did toward the orthodox approach to cancer healing. My purpose was the one of making the change by building; thus by physically creating complementary spaces and I was sufficiently realistic to start feeling my raft overrun by big firms of established 'ergonomic' furniture producers as well as by medical dogmas while rowing against them. Generous enough they would have allowed my little humanistic game, which would not tarnish their way of seeing business as a means for maximum return by perpetuating the distribution of their efficient products.

In both cases, the birth places and the cancer cure, the topic was primarily financial thus political and only consequently cultural. I certainly could have given birth as I would have liked to, but I could not expect to systemically foresee an objective transformation in an apparently and effectively perfectly functioning system.

Furthermore I became aware that my project, unlike the one of other students, was not concerning a way of helping somebody objectively in need of something practical in order to overcome a difficulty or verifiable discomfort. I was not aiming to bring bicycles to African children walking 6 hours on their way back and forth to school, nor was I inventing a system for blind people to be able to safely and independently access street signs and underground networks, as two of my colleague at school were attempting. My project was proposing an improvement to something that was already representing the excellence in our western contemporary world, if anything something so modern and updated as to look forward to.

It was as saying to it: *no thanks*, this perfect system has gone too far and needs to be rebalanced. It was like creating, under the inspiration of my health experience, an organisation aiming at challenging chemotherapy as a cancer cure. Such an orthodox therapy could not be faced and overthrown by the alternative therapies with which I had experimented. After all it had been my personal way of following my nature, feelings and collected information. This only could have broken the *status quo* as a path of misinformation, like the *What doctors don't tell you* magazine was attempting to do.

My approach to birth places was an inside out one, as described in the homonymous co-authored book (5). Why not then create an 'Architecture inside out' centre or Academy where I could teach the principles I had been developing towards a holistic as well as sustainable design?

While figuring out my organization I carried on practising its principles in small consultations in England, providing advice to my mentor as well by applying a specific technique, called Space Therapy(6), in redesigning from the inside out his newly acquired property in Italy. Having made him and his wife very pleased with the proposal, I saw my design passed on, once again, to another professional, the one who had previously drawn up the unsatisfactory nonsense and who would have thus changed his proposal according to mine, and submitted it for approval, of course, with his name. This was justified by my mentor who pointed out that I was a Space Therapist and not an Architect. Incidentally the colleague was not even an architect but, quite obviously, a 'geometra'(7).

The world was going its own way and if ideas such as the ones I wanted to bring forward were going to be exploited even by those who were supposed to coach me toward finding the best way to promote them, which other frustration was I aiming toward? So much care for protecting the bond of mother and child and promoting the 'rooming in' after birth and then, how about my creations? Taken away immediately for good and, at the cheapest rate.

The way out would have been to build an example materializing my ideal approach to the use of space, possibly while teaching and sharing the experience. To do so I had to be my own client or be a catalyst for like-minded people wanting to share a project, that could become the social enterprise I was aiming for.

Despite the fact that the task of the school was to help us to create our own not-for-profit organization, a social venture based on voluntary work and sponsorships derived from other companies' profits, I started by founding, out of my obsessive criticism and certainly out of my habit of earning income through my work, a for profit company based on the fair earnings out of real estate commissions and professional services. The returns were planned to be subsequently conveyed toward a social enterprise to be created in a second stage. I deliberately founded Architecture Inside Out, a limited company, which would also aim for financial returns that would not exclude human and environmental gains, thus would have balanced the former by considering both latter as values to be equally met. I could not but put my heart into the enterprise of which I was the sole director and the sole 'multi-tasked being' which made of course for details to be missed along the way.

Properties to be sold by the company needed to be beautiful, evocative and with character. One of these was an early 19ᵗʰ century *masseria*, a farm located three kilometres from the sea in the Abruzzo Region. It consisted of a block of residential buildings surrounded by seven hectares of land comprising a corn field, olive trees and a one hectare vineyard. Initially I was engaged in consulting the owners about selling it to English investors and then, in visiting, taking pictures, describing it, and offering it to a potential purchaser, interested in dividing it into the highest achievable amount of flats, I decided that I could not possibly allow this to happen. Indeed I had desperately fallen in love with the qualities of the uncontaminated and self contained property, suitable to become a cultural as well as sustainable centre: I was feeling that its identity was specifically gifted and demanding for it to become an agri-cultural centre.

In the meanwhile the company name had changed into Artethis, implying the financial energy to be activated by tuning in with the ones of Art and Ethics, both advocating for beauty, harmony and authenticity as irreplaceable values. Financial resources could then become the capital good, necessary but not sufficient, to increase people, places and community well being by allowing the coming into play of all resources that can help people to cultivate themselves.

The ethical development of the social enterprise that I was aiming for did indeed imply the threefold return; integrating the absolute financial one with the ones of place, history and human beings, complying with the 'triple bottom line' mandate, as I had recently learned. Referring to "people, profit and planet the TBL implies that business can and ought to be run in a financially, socially and environmentally responsible manner". (8)

By focusing on human and environmental assets the idea was to channel the financial ones toward projects that were integrating and adding value to all resources involved. More specifically the explicit aim of the company was the one of enabling individual development through an humanistic use of developments seen as business as well as cultural and educational enterprises inspired by Art and Ethics as regenerating forces for human beings in their wholeness. Believing that people are a combination of spirit and matter and that they are not primarily economic, political and social beings; that everything in the universe is interconnected and that there is more to the world than meet the eye, the company focus was on values and added values pertaining to the wholeness of an evolving humanity, therefore on a use of wealth mindful of context, consciousness and community and in an economy made 'noble' by holistic cultural intentions.

I was projecting my experience and my way of being by seeing the best of people's potential and wishing to contribute towards it. By choosing to identify the company with the spirit of Art and Ethics, I wanted to specify that, in order to create a different and truly innovative scenario, new values, which could only be generated by a new thinking. emphasising the whole rather then the parts, was needed. I was aiming to a shift a new renaissance attempt of resurgence. My own regeneration, confidence and well being confirmed that people's human wholeness was essential and its revaluation crucial to a balanced society. The ideal of beauty and harmony as well as interconnection between past and future, mind activities and craftsmanship, high technology and tradition needed to be manifested.

The *masseria* was offering itself as the perfect context for the first Artethis project. It was comprised of buildings of brick and stone, mellowed by time and weather, embedded in the surrounding countryside and encircled by massive old mulberry and fig trees. The long low line of buildings were in part a private home, with cool vaulted spaces at ground floor and large rooms at the first floor, many vaulted, and with large windows and wrought iron balconies. There were also farm buildings, more recently built, with large doors. Collections of delightful old buildings such as these were already being converted in many parts of Italy into tourist villages, but the idea here was different.

The *masseria* was meant to become a living-working-learning village, where locals and visitors – residents and working people - would create together an environment which was rooted in both local agricultural traditions and the most advanced eco-friendly building techniques. Creating and maintaining a sustainable and eco-friendly environment had become an essential aspect of the project. This would have been achieved by minimizing the consumption and waste of resources and water; preserving and enhancing the ecological features of the land and using natural and recycled materials. In addition, CO_2 and toxic emissions would be considerably reduced via energy-efficient measures and by generating heat and electricity through renewable energy solutions. In short, the aim practically became the one of achieving a healthy and pleasant balance between Nature and People.

The development would consist of the restoration and refurbishment of the existing buildings as well as of the construction of new ones. Both the existing and the new buildings would have residential, private business and communal spaces. The living spaces would consist of a variety of studios, cottages, maisonettes, one-, two- and three -room dwellings – all with kitchens, bathrooms and central heating, and all retaining the original character of the buildings. Some would have vast fireplaces, some vaulted rooms, some balconies, some would be entered by outdoor staircases. Their external appearance would comply with the original. Most units would have had their own private outdoor space.

A limited number of eco-friendly new dwellings would have been located in the surroundings of the existing ones, harmonizing with them.

The purchase price of the poetic place was around one million Euro, equivalent to one of an 80 square meters flat in Santa Margherita Ligure, in the Portofino surroundings, confirmed my brother who immediately jumped at the idea, his presence very valuable, being a financially successful man and also a building administrator.

I liaised between sellers and investors, prepared brochures both in Italian and English, wrote a business plan, designed a scheme, had it quoted, found a qualified restorer who would anticipate all work without any down payment, happy to receive his shares along with the selling of the units, found a company producing the ecological houses open to build the first one upon our project that was almost ready and deliver the following units upon request with a consequent payment during the process without initial disbursement on our part. Eco-consultants joined in from England and a German biomass expert had come to the area and loved the idea of carrying out the first biomass centre in Italy.

The project was multifaceted and complex. For personal reasons the first reliable investor withdrew, one after the other the few others, who would contribute to the purchasing of the property, did the same. The development, in that particular area, was not giving a sufficient return. Tuscany would have been a better area from this point of view! Concrete boxes and traditional flats to be let out at the usual exploitative rate ended up being the obvious observation and choice of most them.

The Ethical Bank, unlike the one in the UK, which would have joined in as partner in such a project, guaranteeing private investors with its presence, would not operate in the same entrepreneurial way in Italy. It declined interest in the enterprise because I was not an immigrant nor a homeless victim, though I would have become one, and because it could not lend money for the purchase and start up of the premises development, which, despite ecology and ethics, was a for profit one. The Italian Ethical Bank would have financed 50% of the enterprise only if I had brought in the English Ethical Bank that turned out not to be inclined in investing abroad.

Green consultants, humanistic builder-restorer, eco-consultants being dropped as a consequence. With a down payment on my part that is still a burden to my body, mind, soul and on my creditors and bank accounts as well, I found myself at a total professional, ideological and personal loss.

In Arezzo, the Community Maternity Centre, that was to include a birth centre, was still not completed after 7 years of the building site for the refurbishment of 1.300sqm. And the worst was that a wall had been built between the community facility area and the birth centre, which I had been informed would never be built.

The birthing pool court case had been won, but the amount of money assessed was not given to me. According to my lawyer, the only way to have it would have been, to promote a declaration of default for the company in my debt, which I did. Meanwhile the company director changed from the Engineer to a Solicitor, bankruptcy law had also changed becoming very disadvantageous for small creditors. In the classical Italian way justice was made to allow 'gentlemen' to ignore duties, and also, I suspect, to allow all the legal boys to play lightly their naughty games. As a conclusion the lump sum agreed without my approval and established by the judge had been sucked by solicitors expenses while the lump in my breast, after seven years, was starting to develop again.

Between the new birthing room furniture there was Symbio, a stool I had designed and redesigned upon the idea of a doctor friend and also named in such a way because of its supportive functions to all interpreters of the birth action. It was going to be distributed by the doctor's son's company after having been produced upon my drawings and under my supervision. After a first pathetic down payment of two thousand Euros for which I had to beg, problems arose that I could not understand, but I perceived these as being excuses not to pay the balance for a change. The selling price of one stool was and is five thousand Euros! Only a letter by an appointed solicitor to whom nobody ever replied and I gave up.

The eco village project collapsed, no financial nor intellectual or emotional rewards from any other jobs or creations, big losses on all my investments and yes 200 Euros as advance payment for the introduction to the revised version of the book *Architecture from the Inside Out* co-authored with Karen Franck. (9)

Bibliography

1 – Dialogues of the Carmelites - opera in three acts by Francis Poulenc. 1953 text George Bernanos. Blanche de la Force becoming sister Blanche of the Agony of Christ.

2 – School for Social Entrepreneurs – London www.the-sse.org

3 – Margaret Sanger (U.S.): Founder of the Planned Parenthood Federation of America, she led the movement for family planning efforts around the world

4 – Dr. Maria Montessori (Italy): Developed the Montessori approach to early childhood education.

5 – Architecture from the Inside Out: From the Body, the Senses, the Site and the Community by Karen A.Franck and R. Bianca Lepori Academy Press; second edition (June 19, 2007)

6 – Space Therapy or The Four Steps to Design Technique that sees design as a way of serving as well as providing a service, being Therapy based on the fourfold meaning of the ancient Greek word 'therapeia' that extends the concept of service to seduction, cure and cult. The Four Steps approach, as Space Therapy, unifies the practical aspects of architecture as service with the more existential ones related to comfort, perception and emotions. For more info see Chapter 4 Space Therapy Bianca Lepori in Architecture from the Inside out. Whiley Academy 2007

7 – geometra :geometer or geometrician. The word composed by the Greek words geo = land and meter= measure indicates the professional ability to measure and value land thus a topographical skill as well as knowledge of building materials, regulations and market.

8 – www.greenmarketingtv_2010_07_05_what-is-a-social-entrepreneur

9 – Architecture from the inside out- ibidem

CHAPTER 6

WHAT AM I DOING HERE?
LOSING ABILITY TO CONFORM AND
LEARNING FROM SHAMANISM

H AVING LOST MONEY, PEOPLE and faith in any possible positive outcome and, after 7 years of remission, my breast started hurting and the lump began to grow again. It did not matter that I understood the mechanics. Yes, I knew of neuropeptides and had found out about *bombesin* (1), the secretion of cancer cells acting back on them and making them multiply. The effects of *bombesin* on the growth of cancer cells were discovered between 1970 and 1985, and the last task of Candice Perth seemed to have been the one of blocking the cancer cell growth factor by using a receptor antagonist, which could cause the tumours to stop dividing. A new peptide pharmacology opposed to the old toxic treatments.

I had been there, in Dr. Perth's and other holistic researchers' theories, I had created my professional dream, lived the dream, the illusion, disillusion and failure, betrayal of myself by myself, more than a wound a grief a mourning for a death, mine; while there I was definitely back in Rome, ejected from one planet to another, mute, an alien in need of anything, with no words, no identity no desire to contribute to anything and yet unable to go back to where I was coming from. I was feeling in exile or in a mental asylum like Camille Claudell (2), abandoned and betrayed by her love and master August Rodin. An old wreck, a body of a more than ever unconscious mind, in oblivion, nowhere, in *caput mundi (3)*, getting worse and worse, lost, patching up my right breast with green clay, which was immediately heated up by the internal fire.

I was feeling polluted. I could not believe it but I knew it could be the end, no energy no money no desire to be well. I was not simply sick again, I was more sick then ever, my entire world having collapsed and not knowing what could be there for me. What could I do with this faith of mine? What was I going to do? What was going on with me? No money for alternative therapies, not even the case to talk to my auric healer who had invited me to take one of her courses. I could not afford it, not even at the discounted price she had kindly offered me. Due to obsessive rigour, for wanting to see things as they should have been instead of as they were, I had ended up not so much rowing against the flow but rather running aground. Why hadn't I stopped then, after the first remission and shifted toward the sharing of my last personal experience rather than constantly attempting to objectively actualize an abstract vision? I had been the living proof of the transformational power of being. Why not focus on that? Which was the fear behind the force?

There was something I needed to prove outside myself and something inside myself I was running away from, as if embodied by a need to be or follow a certain behaviour rather than just simply being. There was also the inability to accept the world and its roles as well as the inability to decide to withdraw from it in a privileged or peaceful and protected niche. I was actually running away from these, from any form of apparent privilege. Voted to sacrifice? There was no way to escape. It was more a matter of concern for the rest, as if carrying the responsibility for a global injustice wrapping up everything, for the nonsense under which was buried our treasure, our sparkle, our power of being, our true nature. Ashamed, upset with myself I was in immense turmoil. Of course I could work but where, and mostly, towards what? Every activity was irrelevant, I had just fallen off a utopia and ended in a nonsensical and, except for the money making task, in a purposeless world.

I did not have the concept of working in order to earn, I could not separate doing something I liked from a job as if a job was an opportunity to learn to share to evolve and there was no job out there for me because there was nothing I wanted do any more, no interest no passion, no beliefs. Had I been a privileged, spoiled person? Somebody who could search explore discover live her passion and thirst through her work? Working as a way of being. Had I been a workaholic then?

No interest was left, not even the illusion I had had of being the social entrepreneur of change. Who could have remembered the world pioneer thinker that my papers and CV were still proving I had been? Empty, lost, with identity problems, clashing with mind set patterns I had been bypassing all my life until then, when they were all suddenly running at me.

All I had rejected, the basics I had always ignored and taken for granted were not any more something I was not interested in, but something everybody had and I did not because I could not afford it. There I was, a geared down engine, engulfed for a wrong interplay of breaks accelerator and clutch. Useless engine, useless coachwork rotting away. Never even thought of going to a doctor, of having an x-ray or a blood test. I was waiting, cornered, trying to help friends to find or sell flats without succeeding, great waste of time without the financial source to advertise or to face the least expenditure. Nobody knew my condition, I was also sort of ignoring it.

I did go back to visit the biologist and her husband though. The computer screen was presenting again a hole in the chest area from which they both deduced there was something wrong concerning my lungs. I did not tell them that I was back with a problematic breast and did not go for the lung scan they had suggested. I could not afford it nor did I want to face the medical field where anyone, by noticing my swallowed breast, would have first thought that I was stupid, as I also felt for different reasons, and second that it was compulsory to operate, to remove everything, which I did not want to surrender to. It was like having a pine cone or, better still, a 7x5cm prosthesis of pumice stone on the upper part of my right breast.

What's next? Death? Very much in a present I could not run away from, I could not envisage a future, not even a tomorrow. No pain, only a grey colour not pale, greyish with a face I could not recognize as mine, blank eyes, getting thinner again, "you see how well these old clothes are still fitting you?" new friends were telling me.

I read that stress produces an acid body and an acid body cannot properly heal itself. Stress had produced cancer again and there was no way I could make my life alkaline, despite the tranquil rhythms within the limits of a basic life style. I could not do anything to help myself but stand still and elaborate my grief, pretending it was not there. After all nobody knew how much energy and passion and beliefs I had put into my lost enterprise.

I was desperately drinking aloe arborescens and keeping the mass as much as possible within the limits of the breast skin. Kilos of clay adsorbing the heat, taking away the flame. A good diet yes, vegetables, no fried food, no yeast, no wine, no no no. Nipple suffocating in between the mass.

After all those years involved in the health care sector, with all my doctor friends, could I have not asked somebody confidentially for help? I far preferred to disappear, shamefully, arrogantly maybe, as if I had been travelling as I had always been. I could have just been pursuing another of the interesting adventures of mine. In a way I was, in a far less glamorous way, a way that nobody would be envious of or listen to.

I helped someone who had enthusiastically introduced my first book on Birth Places more than ten years before, to clear her house in view of a conversion whose project would have been done by me but whose credits and appointment ended up going to somebody else. Kore (4) woman advocating for women's rights and selling my praised professional skill against local geometras once again and builders who, due to local Mafia, might have interfered by preventing or not facilitating the bureaucratic and building process. Hurray! It was not as it is not necessarily that way, but the tribal culture implies to relate to the local socio bureaucratic group expecting the approval not so much on quality but as a favour. As it had happened with the English mentor, the quality was required from an anonymous non-tribal person, kicked out, almost hidden, after the service. *Mannaggia a me*, shame on me and my compulsory creativity!

I was so sophisticated in my expectations from myself and so naïve, unable to cope with role playing games. I was aiming to a different world, I was in a different world and taking so seriously this one I could not believe in.

I was really cornered. What could I do, ask for help from the Church as the Kore woman finally suggested me to do? What do you want from me, Universe? Cleaning stairs or bathrooms as somebody also suggested? I have never been a good cleaner and sorry I was not interested in learning how to become one. I could not be a cleaner nor could I be an architect, though I was one, I could not be a lecturer, nor an archaeological surveyor nor a social entrepreneur, nor a writer, nor an inside out thinker. I could not be anything.

A year was spent in misery, in bereavement, no money, no job, no way to find one, the mass in the right breast growing in the impossibility to afford therapies or vitamins. Helped by new and old friends, put up in sitting rooms sometimes I could, others I would not pay for, exchanging favours, writing a new introduction to Architecture from the Inside Out that had become an academic book and having all products of my creations dispersed in a universe of forgetfulness. It was as if I had never existed before, no past no future, suspended in a foreign limbo, completely powerless, numb, a parasite, me, yes, feeling a parasite.

I have been living as a homeless person, without begging, rather detached, a total outsider. Guilty for the failure, guilty for the money I had borrowed, guilty for having betrayed friends out of enthusiasm and good faith. No more energy, no more trust, no more faith, no more, even if I was living out of it. When I needed a pair of shoes,

I could find them walking back home, walking because without the money to pay for a bus ticket, I could find them on a road side wall, clean, elegant, my size. I could also find money notes on the street, the exact money I remember one evening, to pay for a simple hotel and have a good shower and a peaceful night sleep. I found roses too. Three of them, lying gently on another wall, a higher one, in the very centre of town, just to be collected and brought to the lady who had invited me for supper that night. And when I was starving, yes, that morning I was truly starving, and somebody on a bus pointed out to me a small plastic bag at my feet. It wasn't mine, I said, but stayed on to the end of the line because inside I could see the paper of a well known crackers brand and I could have possibly found some of them in it. Everybody gone off the bus and having picked up the bag, I found within the crackers bag a small package in newspaper wrapping. No crackers, not even a bomb, but eggs, carefully folded in a magazine paper. Yes there were my fresh eggs for lunch. As simple as that. Except for money and job, my survival needs were always fulfilled.

There was much freedom when I could detach myself from place and time, from the *what am I doing here?* (5) and accept the itinerant nature of my journey, the experience of the lonely path of wanderers, without having to be trekking in Nepal, nor travelling across Patagonia, nor sailing down the Volga. It wasn't that trendy though, being in Rome, in the centre of Rome meeting colleagues or friends and the crowds of the Vatican Sistine Chapel tourists let alone the ones aiming to the Coliseum, the amphitheatre where thousands had been murdered to please more than one emperor. Blood was still flowing out of those majestically impressive walls.

Is there anything left I could share in this world? The question was rising again. Yes, there was something I could do: get on and help starving people, help the weakest. How many children were dying of famine every year? Why didn't I go and help them, leave everything behind, bad memories, debts, everything everybody. Why not? How would I survive was then the reply, I was deeply sick and with a few chances of dying of starvation myself.

Desperately trapped without even the money to buy a flight anywhere. So cornered and paralysed that I started to wonder that there might have been a reason for that.

I started to accept the circumstances I ended up in and tried to go beyond them at once. Was that an excuse? After all my suffering had been generated by over caring for an absolute world of perfection of justice that could not be of this world. I did know very well the system and meaning of chakras, the energy centres lying along the spinal column. I did know that the two lower ones, located around the pelvic region and related to the animal kingdom, were moving our planet where everybody was minding his/her own offspring his her own family, tribe, and here in Italy yes, his/her own political party or free masons loggia. Only a few were acting from the human chakras lying along the upper part of the column, where heart and throat are located or from the higher or divine ones positioned at the top of the spine and at the crown of the head. It was rather clear how the primary motivations for human beings were related to the two lower energy centres and how greedily rather than instrumentally possession and wealth were taken. How foolish I had been with my enterprise, how foolish to imagine a change in the financial world of developments without considering first a change, a raising of the energy centres choices were made from.

"Anatomy of the Spirit", the fantastic book and video I had been overwhelmed by over new year 2000 in Florida. Caroline Myss (6) and her explanations, anatomy of the spirit yes, reading and interpreting the chakras and consequent behaviours depending on which chakra the person is rooted in and moving from.

It was all making so much sense to me like the Kabala system that Warren Kenton (7) was passing on from ancient Jewish tradition and that was contextualizing human life in the universe. Wasn't this my main interest when I returned to Italy from London in 1984 because both my parents had died six months one after the other? Where was stored then the tracing paper with the tree of life, including the Hebrew letters that I had been drawing, almost painting as in illumination in my parents' kitchen and from which I had learned so much about the structure of universe and human beings? Psychology and astrology were mapped there in a mathematical system making sense of our life.

What was I expecting? Why had I taken all that for granted and acted as if it was a matter of fact that I could bypass and carry on with my projects? With Artethis I had tried to lift up the financial realm to the heart chakra, or at least filter it with such an energy and fallen down in forgetfulness without control of market roles. Of course I had then lost my professional purpose, it wasn't clear in the first place, I had been playing with double standards. Moving from one dimension and adapting, without adapting, to another.

For some unknown reason the purity of intention was becoming impure along the process and I was starting to find out why, if not as a reason as pattern. Impure was becoming also my social interest, my criticism in defence of the weakest, towards landscape old villages and hamlets because of the hidden agenda, a parameter that could never be met.

If the power of the vision was indeed rooted in the upper chakras, it could not be held there. I was letting it drop down slowly according to audience and market, letting it drop in oblivion while distracted in the search for helpers, partners, supporters who would not share the original motivation but mainly the practical one, which would have been in any case an accomplishment.

I found out that with Artethis I had simply been implementing a pattern I had already enacted with my work in the birthing field, initiated by the desire to create the least possible traumatic environment for a soul coming to earth.

The soul was interesting me. Like the adjective spiritual it was an embarrassing word for me. Too big, too pretentious. Who was I to deal with these matters that, far more than intriguing me, were my true dwelling place? So right had been the Italian publisher of a book

I had translated in early '90 when I was so taken by my worldwide public image of new birth places advocate. 'Peace at last' (8) was the original title, subtitle: the after death experience of John Lennon.

I had found it on the desk of my bedroom in Budapest where I was put up by Julia Lazlo, a friend who had very much promoted the book channelled by Jason Leen who had consequently become its author. She had already translated it into Hungarian and was pressing me to do the same in Italian. As author of a rational manual that had de-constructed and reconstructed a model for Birth Places, I was sort of prevented from doing so. Conflicting images, more than interests.

The translation would have invalidated the logic I had imbued all my work with. The book was fascinating and needless to say I utterly enjoyed translating it after having found the Italian publisher for it. Translation completed I felt that I would not mix my visionary professional identity with the 'unorthodox and unprofessionally' visionary one of the Lennon book and proposed the anagram of my name as official translator to the publisher by whom I had been appointed because of my name, as author of a book on Birth Places. Surprised and disappointed he asked me to enquire into my suggestion, inviting me to have the courage of manifesting my beliefs. Having ignored the book ever since, I rediscovered it on the occasion of a visit to Rome of Jason Leen himself, in 2008, when I had found out that the title "Peace at last" had become: L'energia dell'amore: John Lennon messaggero di luce (9), The energy of love: John Lennon messenger of light, translated by . . . me, with my actual name. I was so pleased then to have turned out being officially the translator!

It became clear what I had done wrong, what I was doing wrong. The rational part of me was understanding, I could not be but black or white, choosing the white, by name and by intention and acting as black, ending up grey or beige, champagne or magnolia, so classic and anonymous, so adaptable as background.

I was feeling a crawling, creeping grovelling thinking cornered worm.

There wasn't any indication toward a way out until the Teacher of Lucid Dreams, a book by Olga Karithidis (10), was lent to me by Veronica.

There, on the 9th floor where I was lucky enough to be nourished by a very strictly naturalist retired Alitalia stewardess, I dived non stop into the presented kindred experiences images and sentences.

You do not have to fight the discomfort, you must let it develop and follow it . . . you can not walk on the rope if you are afraid. (11)

Blanche de la Force. Which force?

The setting was Siberia, a far away environment of remote cultures, prior to the Western predictable mental order and roles. A place of not necessarily religious rituals where Shamanism, as it was before Christianity, before communism and capitalism was practised, as Dr. Karitidis, a psychiatrist described in her adventurously professional journey in Samarcanda, where she had been initiated by the Teacher of Lucid Dreams. A cultural shift, which integrated her practice with shamanistic disciplines and made of her a healer, implying healing at its purest form.

We are not responsible for the pain other people have produced in us, it is not our fault if we have been wounded and it is not us who need to be ashamed of this.(12) If you allow such a pain to crystallize in your memory, as a non resolved knot, it will transform itself in the incubator, in the womb in which the malignant and hungry spirit, which had remained posted in your genetic memory, will get strength and nourishment and will poison your existence. (13)

Spirits of the trauma, I was reading, were created every time something was hurting us without our accepting it. People seem to recreate traumas in the attempt to ask for help, which was possibly my case. But what was the original trauma? By using time as a partner, it was suggested in the book, difficulties and conflictual experiences were eventually meant to transform themselves into knowledge. Time, I seemed to have plenty in my everyday routine, but also not enough due to the gigantic lump and terrible shape, let alone the financial difficulties I was in.

Having just worked out my pattern of falling from higher chakra vision to market application in my professional practice and social enterprises, I came across another sentence, a metaphor, an image, that instantly pointed out where I had always felt I was coming from.

When the acrobats walk on the rope, their space transforms itself, in such a moment they do not think of living on the earth but believe of being creature of the sky, they live in the sky and make a visit on earth, as if they would arrive in the past from a place of the future, they transform the past of people who are watching them while bringing the energy of the future.(14)

This was it, my joy, my fulfilment, but there then I was feeling in the past and desperately missing the energy of the future. What was I waiting for? I had it, only needed to regain and better utilize it, but for some reason it was as if I had lost the spring, I could not get to it. Had I buried it, sealed with the rock of my fears? Which fears?

Remember the three acrobats? I was reading, *If you are one of the two who are sitting and it is somebody else taking them up to that height you are powerless. You can have the control of the situation only when you are the tight rope walker, the perceiver. At eyes level there is no memory but perception. Become the observer and nothing will be missed. When you experience sadness it means that the trauma is rooted on an action or non action of yours that had produced a wound. In order to start healing you have to activate an opposite process: you have to heal the memory by working on perception. (15)*

The weight of non action seemed to be far heavier than the one of wrongly taken actions. And then there was all my activity which was not action but excuse for action. Who was that other self I was - not aware of - who had forced me to move in circles, possibly around a wound, instead of turning shoulders to it and positively moving on?

No energy for detecting that deeper wound, nor the demon living inside me.

The powerful images of the acrobats, the ones of dreams were key to access a particular space of memory that was always related to another space. Their main purpose being, according to the Teacher of Lucid Dreams, the one of compensating for the leaks of our memory in order to defeat the demons. I could verify how in my own experience, I was indeed not sad because of the unsuccessful Artethis enterprise, which had been only the superficial image connecting me to my space of pain. There was something in the project, as it had been on my birth prototypes, that was acting as a key of memory from which my sadness would spring. Indeed it was not Artethis nor the failure I was feeling miserable for.

After Zoroaster having separated everything in black and white, consciousness has been removed from the centre of existence. (16)

In my book and lectures I had been using left and right brain functions diagrams with the aim of detecting forms and materials that would be appropriate to specifically dedicated environments. Between the left brain traditional hospital delivery room and the right brain home birth, my aim was the one of pointing out how a new type, emerged from my research and interviews was needed as a synthesis of the two, in view of a natural birth, considered safe because it was in a hospital environment. Although opposite, the two hemisphere functions would be active simultaneously and switch from one to the other flexibly. Why then separate them so rigidly in our physical creations, missing out on the excluded parts all the time?

While I had seen the synthesis between the two hemispheres of the cerebral cortex in the band of nerve fibres called *corpus callosum*, here was the Teacher resolving the problem of the asymmetry between the two hemisphere's functions, thanks to the cerebellum or little brain, able to coordinate relationships because of the many neuronal connections it is composed of. Rather than being considered, as it is by the scientific world, a system responsible for the moving coordination, the little brain was coming to be understood as the coordinator point of imagination, dreams and memoires. Rather than keeping consciousness at the cortex level, exercises have indicated moving it to the basis of the skull where the little brain was becoming the pivot of a new consciousness.

Needless to say I had tried to focus as suggested and experimented with the visualisation of a swastika, a very powerful symbol, considered to be able to resolve the problem of the division of our psyche, its arms connecting present and past, action and perception, its centre being related to all places of memory. A symbol acting as bridge towards undivided time.

Bibliography

1 – Bombesin from Candace Perth Molecules of emotion The science behind Mind-Body Medicine Simon & Schuster; first edition September 1997

2 – Gérard Bouté *Camille Claudel: La Miroir et la Nuit.* Les Editions de L'Amateur

3 – *Caput mundi* Latin expression dating back to the time of the Imperial Historian referring to Rome as capital of the world as it was then known

4 – Kore a psychological aspect, the Persephone girl, equivalent to Pan

5 – What am I doing here- Bruce Chatwin Penguin (Non-Classics); Second edition edition (August 1, 1990)

6 – Carolyn Myss Anatomy of the Spirit: The Seven Stages of Power and HealingThree Rivers Press; 1 edition (August 26, 1997)

7 – Warren Kenton English name of Z'ev Ben Shimon Halevi Kabbalah Tradition of Hidden Knowledge Thames & Hudson (1985)

8 – Peace at last – The After-Death Experience of John Lennon by John Lennon and Jason Leen Illumination Arts Publishing Company (February 1, 1998)

9 – L'energia dell'amore : John Lennon messaggero di luce Jason Leen – Macro Edizioni 1999

10 – Olga Kharitidis The master of lucid dreams: Hampton Roads Pub Co (December 1, 2001
11 – ibidem
12 – ibidem
13 – ibidem
14 – ibidem
15 – ibidem
16 – ibidem

CHAPTER 7

TIFERET, THE PLACE OF BEAUTY BETWEEN EARTH AND SKY: REMEMBERING KABBALAH

" THE SHE SHAMAN" (1) WAS the second book by Olga Karitidis, borrowed as soon as I had finished her first. Equally intriguing the description of the author's meeting and her healing experience with a lady intermediary between the human and the spirit world; a woman of very strong powers, whose approach to illness consisted in restoring peoples' individual balance by entering the supernatural dimension. Directed by spirit guides, possibly in trance, her body *weaving between states of consciousness and unconsciousness,(2)* she would eliminate the physical or psychological ailment by freeing people from the spirit of the trauma.

Shamanism in Siberia had been persecuted and shamans put in jail, by Communists and Catholics alike, because of their personal access to the spiritual world and because of their assumed primitive beliefs and cultural backwardness compared to Western science. For these reasons, the old woman was living in solitude, away from the village of Altaj, in an ordinary green painted house surrounded by a wooden fence, and plenty of snow in winter time.

More than remarkable, she was at least seventy years old, wearing a long skirt made of different types of differently coloured fabrics. She had little dolls hanging on her back and dark hair under a blue scarf. I imagined her dancing as described, accompanied by drums, in an almost masculine warrior like duel. I could imagine the fire at the centre of the room where her rituals would have taken place and the dark wooden table covered by dust, like everything, including the carpets on the floor where therapies on naked bodies would be performed. An ancestral environment for an off limits experience in which bodies could even be scratched and hands tied up to wall bolted rings. An extreme experience, as I was feeling my condition was.

Having lost, like the author, any trust in doctors, I would have made every attempt for that woman in Siberia to be able to get hold of my spirit of the trauma and make me free of it.

Healing seamed to imply a fight, not against disease, but against a part of ourself. No compassion, no politeness then, no comprehension for the demon of the trauma that needed to be fought in a rough tough head-on body collision, taken to the extreme end close to the boundary of physical death.

Possibly facing physical death in such a primitive and violent way could have helped overcome inner conflicts. I was longing for a shocking experience that would make all my thoughts fall silent, for *the smile of an endearing, miracles performing, crazy old lady.(3)*

My life was following the usual routine, including buying every month a bottle of aloe syrup, made by a Jesuit brother, gardener very knowledgeable about medical plants, herbs and natural remedies. My pattern had always been the one of quickly collecting the remedy and disappearing as soon the bottle was handed to me by the brother. One evening he had been caught in traffic and for the first time I did not find him waiting for me. Wondering about how to contact Olga Karitidis and how to dissolve into a primordial order, aware that it would have been impossible for me to go anywhere anyway and being very weak, without even making the choice of staying or leaving, I sat down in the waiting room of the monastery for an indefinite length of time.

Once arrived, the almost ninety year old brother, apologized for the delay and for the first time, probably because I was sitting there and certainly because of my grey face, he asked what my problem was.

BIANCA LEPORI

After my reply, with a shaky soft voice "I don't know", he added, "but, I have recently met a woman who is dissolving cancer and does not want to be paid". Soon I found out that, from where I was living, I could reach her by tube and bus in half an hour.

Her face was beautiful, soft smooth skin, green eyes, long light chestnut hair, tied loosely at the nape. Looking at me on the opposite side of the dining table, she was smiling with control and indifference as she was at least thinking if not seeing something she could not share. She did not say a word when she saw my pinecone-like right breast: only started massaging with warm oil. Before leaving I had my first coffee after years and in the afternoon, at home, her phone call: "How are you feeling?" There were only red spots on the skin where she had been massaging, a sort of rush.

The following morning the mirror showed a new light in my eyes. I went up to my Siberia again, another massage, another coffee, another rush, terrible smell when leaving the loo and back to my face in a very short time. Every morning, except for weekends, I climbed up to that part of the city, located North of the Vatican and dotted with religious institutes. Developed in the 60's my healer's neighbourhood specifically was characterized by streets named after popes and cardinals. A non orthodox shamanistic environment, but there she was, isolated behind that turquoise blue gate, in an ordinary big house with its broad front garden with flower beds separated by gravel paths; a gold fish pond and the pomegranate tree just outside her front door, on its left hand side.

"Buongiorno germoglio", she used to welcome me. I was flourishing and she was calling me sprout. After each treatment she would disappear into her huge kitchen that reminded me of the Siberian shaman's environment. Not exactly aseptic like the huge sitting room and its far too long table, possibly five meters long, where her oil and cotton wool were laid over an old plastic tablecloth. Coffee was served in two tiny porcelain cups tightly positioned on a little metal tray, far too small, almost a cute dolls set, on such a vast table.

I remember flying away from her house after each treatment, leaving at my shoulders her gate and walking towards the bus stop along the one way street, named after a cardinal I could only imagine as severe and unfriendly like his terribly cacophonous name. An ordinary road of non historical surroundings, ordinary concrete buildings, beige-brown ordinary design handrails with ordinary shops, a small food supermarket and a bakery, a flower shop, a coffee bar and patisserie, a lottery kiosk, a smoking lady tobacconist and a newsagent. A shot of suburban soulless chaos, an invitation for the eyes to blind themselves, which I did while taken by a psychological unwinding, difficult to explain.

Progressively, with the melting away of the mass, I was becoming free from the events that had generated it. It generally happened when leaving her house, it was like going back for a second in the memory of the flesh, having a glimpse of an episode and letting it go forever without holding on to it, without reviewing it, discussing it.

After these peaks of awareness, the very deep process, triggered by the treatment, was taking up most of my day. The price for freedom. A few tears sometimes on the street, the amazing experience being uniquely mine.

A miracle for the way, the how, the synchronicity with the shaman book and my projections. I was getting well, feeling well. My breast emptying. "Where does the lump go?", she asked. "Washed out with faeces", we laughed. Gone indeed as I could see from my face, my energy and vivacity.

She was wearing family jewels that had become part of her body, a ring, a bracelet and a necklace with pendants, one of which was an amulet that she insisted saying was a child, hanging on her décolleté rather than on her back, as in the case of the Siberian lady. An elegantly designed thick red golden snake with tie and muzzle bent each to the side of a big dark stone, lid of a portrait holder as hardly detected from the fine hinge on one of the stone sides. The snake that, according to the ancient Greek tradition was seen as a healer and that, by the Siberian shaman, was considered as the image of one's own power, possibly a key to complete a healing process. *Hold it in your hands,* she suggested, *and remember the sensation of having to find the balance between yourself and this power you are holding. If you keep it too tight the snake might bite you. If you do not keep it tight enough you will loose hold of it and you will miss out. (4)*

Find the right balance and maintain it. She, my Italian shaman, had been able to use it. With herself, her children and the nursing home she had been running. She was not a mystic, but indeed *a woman who could do anything she wanted, easily and fast . . . who had done anything anybody else had done but she was . . . more courageous than most people are . . . somebody who works hard to keep alive those who want to pass away.(5)*

The snake. I was looking at it sometimes, while wondering where had my power gone. Did I keep it too tight and it had bitten me or did I not keep it tightly enough and I had lost it? Which power are we talking about here? Whose power? I never wanted power, I despised power. Still I had been deeply affected by another shaman's words I had taken note of years before while watching a movie. In the film Wolf (6), the priest-doctor reveals and confirms, to a brilliantly performing Jack Nicholson in the process of becoming a wolf after having been bitten by one such an animal, the instinctive quality he will inherit from it : *power without fear, love without doubt.*

It took my healer three months to completely melt the pumice mass, relieve the pain in both sides of my chest, from arm pits down to just above the waist. Her hand was drawn towards the part whose illness I had not yet become aware of: by pressing a particular area, the pain was emerging and one layer after the other, one session after the other, she was taking it away, removing it from its source, almost by aspirating and absorbing it. The pain was unbearable and the fear even more so. The idea that the cancer could have entered my ribs was truly terrifying me. I asked her about this, but she was negative about it. The pain was disappearing and I was enchanted.

Life was again flowing through me, cleaned despite the un-hygienic environment. I was feeling so blessed for the experience, so privileged for having trusted enough to be trusted, for having been helped once again to defeat death. Anything else was ridiculously redundant and there was the thrilling thought of being extremely poor but so rich at once to overcome practical difficulties with no objections nor complaints. No explanation either about my new health, it did happen. No xray before or after. No reports nor documentation. Whom do I have to give a demonstration to? It was only a matter between myself and myself.

A couple of weeks by the sea, tanned and healthy again. Free from the lump and from the daily commitment. "I'd like to have a check up on you", she rang after having had a dream. Having gone back to her, she found that full remission had not happened: something very painful was resisting and beginning to spread again around my right arm pit.

Fall 2007. In remission again and convalescent from life I moved back to the office I had left 7 years before. I needed to start from somewhere, mainly to put together some money. I did not start for a job but for a space to work in and from, a section of an articulated desk offered by a colleague: my computer and familiar working atmosphere. Sometimes a vague instinct toward joining a team, a group that in Italy could not be but political: housing, community services, mixed use of space, an inside-out practice about the use of land, that would have interested me in an artistically and environmentally blessed country with the worst possible speculation and land abuse. Not the least hint of architecture, solicitors involved in the development field, financial consultants, nothing new in the chasing of the 6.5% return at least in commercial investments, a real estate sector far more devastated than I could have envisaged while founding Artethis: white collar estate agents ignoring any sense of space, orientation, aesthetics, considering ethics a fashion brand. Environmental criminals, resources given to a back-warding, stuffy, obsolete, corrupt, repetitive, a-meritocratic, chauvinistic system, a genitally and belly driven one, not even a hint towards raising energy above the diaphragm. Heart mentioned on valentine's day over a chocolate box or in emotionally manipulative trash TV programs. No proposals, never, only unavoidable critics of a system of lobotomised brains. Intercessions, always, *padrini* always, in business or religion, lover priests, loving Magdalenes.

Teaching became my resource, some Italian for foreigners but mainly English for Italian students. I was enjoying coordinating the lessons and particularly reading the English literature and history I had never studied before. The dislike for ecclesiastical privilege was not only fascinating to me but I experienced it almost physically as a relief from a burden. Questioning the church's behaviour and doctrines was a topic I was feeling particularly attracted to. I identified with Wycliff (7) attacking the Church's wealth and properties as well as the sinful priests and bishops, considered outside god's law, and questioning their presumed ability to transform bread into the body of Christ. After Wycliff's ideas came the deep breath of rigorous clarity of the Lollards' movement (8) profoundly against church political positions, confusing the matter of the State with the matter of the Spirit: so remarkable and contemporary in a world of hypocrisy and complicity. So interesting also the idea, not indicated in the schools texts but found in my research, about their adoption of the metempsychosis doctrines imported from France by those few Cathars who succeeded in escaping the persecution of the Inquisition and joining the British community.

Guest in the office without practising, but sheltered and part of a team, suggesting, consulting when asked. Meeting my healer once or twice a week, her wild informality so much more real than many appearance games. Such a very strong woman, aristocratic by family, informal, very self contained, a world apart, with the flavour of the South, of the land she was born in, a big family of land owners with deep roots in the ground, very religious mother and less religious father, a fat priest often visiting their home, "but when will he give birth" she was asking her parents, imagining a little darkly dressed priest eventually coming out of don Antonio's belly.

Vivacious, far too, riding a horse in the village when adolescent, escorted by two of her brothers, one on each side, sitting on the front row in the class where her jealous husband taught Greek, yes, taken to school by her jealous husband/father to listen to his classes. She had never gone to school, only private lessons, at home. Still incredibly vivacious despite a painful knee, a generous woman, mother and grandmother, informal, totally informal, ready to be and go where she was needed.

Over 70, she was wearing a raffle flounced old fashion long skirt, each flounce often of different materials, in different nuances of the same colour. How many stories I had heard from her past her dreams, lucid in her own way, often flying above earth or encountering difficulties, entities intervening and removing the key of the car she was driving while committed to healing somebody very dear to her she was not by others allowed to. Not easy her life, people not always understanding nor supporting her gift far beyond their understanding. *'You are from another planet'* she loved it so much when I said it to her. Listening to me sometimes, too seldom, almost afraid to.

How much I would have liked to talk to her, to confront her power with the one of other healers, to pin her down to the fact that her healing power, yes, could have been directly from God, as she said, but other people could have had a similar one. How could she have confronted herself? Her big eyes were intrigued by the idea of being a channel of god, the non discussable being nobody wanted to challenge but honour in all its forms and more.

It could have been a gift, she could have been, she was a channel, a broker, an intermediate between one world and another, but I could not say, I could not tell her about all my previous healing experiences, my wonders, nor about the shaman I wanted to visit in Siberia when finally I ended up meeting her. Or may be she could have, but I did not say anything.

So religious, so Christian, in a network of nuns and priests, surrounded by images of Jesus and padre Pio, rosaries and Virgin Mary's and small altars. So Christian and so pagan, so informed and disillusioned about the Church, the celibacy cabaret, the Vatican properties, not so much informed about the only – fiscal - paradise on earth, the IOR, (9) the Vatican bank and its international intrigues and victims.

She listened to my criticism, adding her own. No charity from the church she knew very well: when there was a critical case, when there was a mentally ill or difficult person, nuns would call her and drop the person at her home for a short time that would never end. She was generous but she could not stand the idea of so many floors she knew being vacant in the monasteries where the difficult cases were coming from. 'We can't keep them' was apparently the reply of the obedient nuns, orienting their commercial trend toward holiday homes, a straightforward business for not necessarily holy days in Rome.

So critical and yet so unavoidably bolted into a mind both very generous and ego suffocating, brushing out other people's creativity, mine as well, the one I could have shared together with my trying to make sense of my life process, to feel part of a design rather than simply of a contradictory fantasy alimented by authorities not walking their talk. There was a conflicting link and more than once I wondered about our personal karmic one.

My immediate and crucial purpose was the making up for the lost money that would at least take away the constant financial stress. It was clear that I was lacking context. I was de-contextualized. *Perdersi, l'uomo senza ambiente*(10) was the title of an interesting social science book of the '90s. *'Loosing oneself, man without context'*. Having lost all coordinates in Rome and in my country, my terrain wasn't related to my history and I often identified myself with that book title. I had ended up in a religious circuit I did apparently had anything to do with. The cultural level of the country was *terrificante*, a word not equivalent to the English terrific, which in Italian would have been *fantastico*, but too appalling. Calendar woman imposed as Minister of Equal Opportunities between men and women, an ordinary 'primary school teacher' like young lady appointed as Minister of Education. Everyday offences to the intelligence and slashes to the dignity and to a true contribution of the feminine to society. Minister of Culture the dolphin of the uncultured, more cultured indeed of the ex butcher, appointed as coordinator of the People of Freedom, the leading Italian political party, generating hate between North and South and racial discrimination, despite the additional self given epithet of 'Party of Love'.

The prince Prime Minister manipulating the country through his own media and escaping any possible trial through purposely formulated laws aimed to protect him from jail, including the abrogation of the crime for balance sheet falsification. I was ashamed to be Italian. Sex and money,

money and sex, cars, yes and football indeed, money, sex, cars and lies, television, metaphorical abuse, literal abuse, lies, confessions, complicity, scandals, barbarities with the purpose of possessing, buying cars and sex and having the money for bribery, corruption and abuse and insane behaviours in a Roman catholic country.

What am I doing here? Right wing or Left wing parties, opposites in values but equal in unconsciousness. Acquisitive in a different way, pessimistic, genetically catholic, non holistic, oppositional, always. I am good and you are bad, you are bad and I am good, you are bad and I am doing the same, on a different scale, I overcharge when I have to get, I complain when you get, when she gets and I do not. Mine is mine, mine is not yours, rights yes rights. Duties when? Recycling money by buying real estates or building new developments was the main entrepreneurial activity of the country involving solicitors, accountants and notaries, the institutional granters of legality in transactions.

Not a clue about architecture or urban design: a scheme of linear buildings promoted and accepted each one as a new town, without a square, not even a proper sewage system, nor a bus stop or connection with L'Aquila, the town of which they were supposed to be satellites after the destruction that occurred in the April 2008 earthquake. Propaganda for the prince hiding behind empty words the affairs of his closest collaborators after financial recognition for their complicity.

In which country I wondered could there have existed a party lead by a mass manipulator and called 'People of freedom' as if it were the people and their freedom that mattered? A disguised dictatorship masterpiece, a democratic paradox, a social absurdity, a burial of the intelligence. Cancer is also this. It is politics, it is a prime minister offending and further manipulating masses that had voted for him under the slogan 'we shall beat cancer too' with crowds of eunuchs, women and men alike, all clapping together. A country prone to manipulation, to anything but inner freedom and consciousness. What am I doing here?

A native cultured immigrant from inside the EU. Speechless, retired without a pension, only a pedigree. More than a successful failure, a failed success. Living in a 'basso' kindly offered by a friend for a cheap rate, humid, dark, uninhabitable by standards, but rented out, why not, we are in the centre of Rome and Rome is Rome, there will always be somebody ready to rent anything next the Coliseum. Left wing, an exploitative attempt I had to be grateful for.

Mould, fungus, darkness, often wandering about, anywhere, particularly in day time, particularly on week ends. Waking up with electric light, the only glazed panel being a French window opening on to the street, a very bohemian one indeed, with no cardinal nor popes nor bishops name, with typically Roman sepia and terracotta red painted buildings walls and three white Corinthian columns standing out at one of its ends, an archaeological screen, almost as if they were a *trompe l'oeil*.

Left over furniture inside the studio flat, copper pipe falling out of its supporting brackets, an unloved and unlovable Chinese lamp hanging down from the ceiling. Left over of very badly matching plates, glasses, cups, cutlery badly combined. A collection of un-aesthetic cheapness. What am I doing here? Where is the style, the harmony and where are the exceptionally tasteful chosen objects, at almost zero cost, I had always been surrounded by?

I needed to breath oxygen but also beauty. I needed to smile over a line, to reduce the realm of my vision into a face a flower a leaf a jewel a stone. I could no longer be indifferent to carelessness and ugliness because they were irritating me, experiencing the latter in particular as deformation of the divine, as heartless manifestation of heartless souls. I was in Italy paradoxically feeling surrounded by ugliness, becoming ugly myself, making myself sick, again.

Tiferet was the name I could not ignore, there on the front window of the shoes shop I was passing by on the way back from my healer. Intrigued by the shoes but more by the name, which means beauty in Hebrew and which was sending a specific message to my soul. Tiferet, yes, there, where I liked and needed to be, the place of beauty, truth, harmony and compassion in the Tree of Life, the Kabbalah diagram illustrating the pathway of Divine emanation in its journey of consciousness from the eternal life, EIN SOF OR, down to Malkut, the material world and back again from this to the higher realms.

As if I had died as if I had all forgotten, now in a new life, in this life, remembering again almost as if after a new birth. The Tree of Life as I had learned about it, at first, in Jerusalem from Adin Steinsaltz's book The Thirteen Petalled Rose.(11) *"The physical world in which we live . . . is only a part of an inconceivable vast system of worlds. Most of these worlds are spiritual in their essence, they are of a different order from our own world . . . The various worlds inter-penetrate and interact in such a way that they can be considered counterpart of one another, each reflecting or projecting itself on the one below or above it" (12)*

In the Kabbalistc tradition the worlds are four and represent different dimensions of being, from light to matter, through energy and form. Each of them is defined according to a geometrical pattern consisting of ten Sefirot, forces or channels of divine flow emanating from Keter, the crown or divine will, down to Malkut, the kingdom. Tiferet is one of the ten Sefirot.

It was thanks to the lectures and workshop of Warren Kenton in London integrating the wisdom of the tradition with a graphic representation that I could visualize the concepts previously grasped in Jerusalem and experience the geometry of each world, the effectiveness of the Tree of life and the meaning of each Sefira. Having trained as an architect and inspired by ancient drawings pertaining to the Kabbalistic tradition, Kenton was delineating on paper the structure of each world, the mechanics of how the ten Sefirot interrelate and how the four worlds interlock, offering in a 'meta-design' (13) format, the construction of the visible and invisible universes as well as a map for the soul.

Once upon a time, *before the Beginning, there was, is, and always will be EIN SOF, the Divine field of eternal formlessness. Within the EIN SOF, a yearning arose, a yearning for 'Face to gaze upon Face;' EIN SOF wished to behold itself, so it withdrew itself from one place. A void appeared ". . . in which the mirror of existence could be manifested." (15)*

EIN SOF OR, Eternal Light, surrounded the void and emanated into it, manifesting ten distinct qualities or energies,the ten Sefirot. (16)

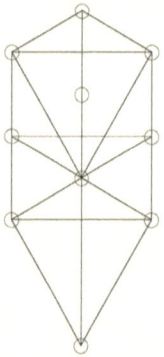

From
Z'ev ben Shimon Halevi

During the Sixth phase, the sixth Day of Creation, the Divine emanation unfolded into the Four Worlds of Emanation (Azilut), Creation (Beria h), Formation (Yetzirah), and Manifestation (Assiyah), with the ten energies (Sefirot) unfolding in each world manifesting in ten different energies or Sefirot. (17)

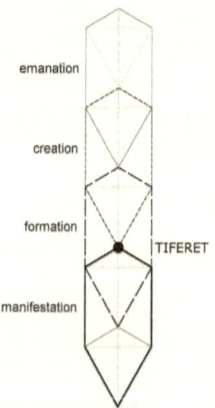

From
Z'ev ben Shimon Halevi

Thanks to the Kenton theory and graphics the tree of life from metaphysical had become physical and the four interlocking worlds, identical to the first one, started to naturally slide visually down from the higher world to the lower one along the three illustrated pillars, the central of which being the one of balance. It became understandable and clear then that, along this pillar, the top apex of the fourth world of manifestation coincides with the bottom apex of the second world of creation, there where the world of matter meets the world of spirit. That place of connection between the higher and lower worlds is Tiferet, at the heart of the third world of formation, which is the one of form where we are located as human beings, between matter and spirit.

Being that the diagram is a sacred map expressing universal principles related to the Macrocosm of existence and influencing individual human beings, we, as microcosms, are built upon the same template thus on an identical tree that is composed, on its own turn, of four worlds relating to the individual rather than to the cosmic and the collective

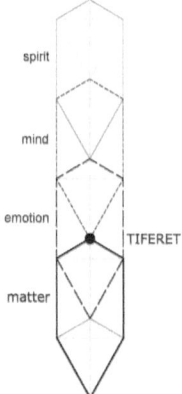

From
Z'ev ben Shimon Halevi

Since a Living Being (Human Being) was created and formed in the image of the Tree of Life the Tree of Life lived within the Being and mirrored the Tree of Life in all The Four Worlds; with the ten energies (Sefirot) unfolding in four levels of being: Spirit, Mind, Emotion, and Matter.(17)

97

In the tree of human beings Tiferet, at the point of connection between the worlds of Matter and the one of Mind is at the heart of the second world of Emotion, which is overlapping both of them. It is the place of Harmony as combination of Beauty, Truth and Compassion. Including matter it is the place of the soul along the central pillar, which in the human tree is the one of consciousness. There where, according to Kenton, action emotion and intellect cohere (18), and where, according to Steinsaltz, there is a moral as well as aesthetic acceptance of the world (19), there where I was longing to be, where unconsciously I attempted to go with Artethis LTD.

This will always be my preferred tale, the one I knew and had always been longing for, the one that helped me to locate myself in the universe. The answer to what am I doing here is in understanding where I am there, within and along the tree, a combination of ancient teachings and modern knowledge, having zigzagged down, as a particle of eternal light, to Malkutt, our anchor point to the earth, the lower world of matter.

A descent with consequent loss of remembrance and the ascent towards awareness while, the *power of containment, balance, and expansion still exists in all of us. We have only to reclaim our inheritance of divinity, and our birthright of eternal life, to manifest again our ascension to wholeness. Each human who recognizes this spark of divinity within and is willing to create unity with their soul, reclaims this power. We have descended to the furthest and densest frequencies in the universe and now it is time for our return to wholeness (20)*

Bibliography

1 – The She-Shaman, Italian title for Entering the Circle : A Russian Psychiatrist's Journey into Siberian Shamanism Olga Kharitidi Gloria Press; 1st edition October 1995

2 – ibidem

3 – ibidem

4 – ibidem

5 – ibidem

6 – Wolf.- film Mike Nichols 1994

7 – John Wycliff (1320-1384) was a theologian and early proponent of reform in the Roman Catholic Church during the 14th century. He initiated the first translation of the Bible into the English language and is considered the main precursor of the Protestant Reformation http://www.greatsite.com/timeline-english-bible-history/John-wycliffe.html

8 – The Lollards. Followers of John Whycliff founders of the political and social movement called Lollardy. http://en.wikipedia.org/wiki/Lollardy

9 – IOR (Istituto per le Opere di Religione) the so called Vatican Bank.

10 – Perdersi L'uomo senza ambiente Franco La Cecla – Laterza 2005

11 – Adin Steinsaltz – The Thirteen petalled Rose – A discourse on the essence of Jewish existence and belief- Basic books, inc, Publishers New York 1980

12 – Adin Steinsaltz – The Thirteen petalled Rose page 3

13 – 'Meta-design' intended as the functional diagram of functions and relationship upon which design will be based

14 – Warren Kenton English name of Z'ev ben Shimon Halevi Kabbalah Tradition of Hidden Knowledge Thames & Hudson (1985)

15 – ibidem

16 – ibidem

17 – ibidem

18 – ibidem

BIANCA LEPORI

19 – Adin Steinsaltz – The Thirteen petalled Rose page 61
20 – Kenton English name of Z'ev ben Shimon Halevi Kabbalah
Tradition of Hidden Knowledge Thames & Hudson (1985)

CHAPTER 8

THE SPREADING OF THE DISEASE: GOING DEEPER INTO HEALING BY LEARNING FROM PREVIOUS LIVES

M Y DESCENT INTO DARKNESS did not end nevertheless nor had I the time to accommodate the recollection. After one year in the 'basso', literally down where I had fallen, the dampness had been devastating. My body again, my chest swallowed, I could hardly breathe. I was coughing, my heart suffocating, it was impossible to walk up a flight of stairs without wondering if I could make it. No breath at all. I could not ask again for help, again for free After so much had been given.

You may simply need your energy to be realigned, why not go to the young woman I have recently met? She has literally been transforming the energy of the people she has treated". "What does she do?" "I do not know but I know that it works" were Veronica's words. Of course I would meet the person she had suggested.

The new lady, living outside Rome, an hour away, was also living in a secluded place. She must have been 25 years old, a girl's face, dressed in white, heavily pregnant. In a dialogue before starting, she anticipated that her treatment would last between 30 and 40 minutes. Lying on her massage bed I could imagine her working on my head and then moving towards my chest. Five minutes all together, not more and she left. Already done? When she returned she said she was sorry she could not treat me, that she was pregnant and had been instructed not to work on my body, particularly on my chest. Another short dialogue, "I know only one person who can help you, he lives in Milan, this is his book, this is his phone number, it may take a couple of years to have an appointment.

I had my splendid healer and went back to her, chest, right and left breast, lungs, coughing more than ever, stomach, ovaries and kidneys. Pain was everywhere. As she was pressing a point a new pain would emerge as soon as the upper layer was dissolved. Two treatments a day, one in the evening and one in the morning, early morning reason for which I spent the night at her place, awakened early, after being unable to sleep until too late. She was nervous, concerned, tense for the never ending process that this time was taking up all her energy. The pain on both sides of my chest and the fear of cancer having reached the bones," No it is only clung to them, she could see, "it is like having an ex ray of your under skin lying on this table" were her words.

"Lo caccio"- I am going to chase it away. She was pressing, particularly on my ribs, always finding deeper layers of intolerable pain, I was afraid, my bones, the lungs, coughing, coughing out all suffocated dampness, piles of tissues with mucus that everyday she removed through my nose. Disgusting mucus, more and more of that one too, a never ending unusable quarry. Tired, concerned dependant, upset for dependence and grateful. Spotting metastasis as if they were a magnet, she was pressing the point-area first and then keeping her hand a few centimetres above the flesh, tingling was the signal. Absorbing the pain, dissolving the congested mass.

In one or more sessions pain would disappear. My chest became looser, my lungs more openly breathing, but still coughing. I will never forget how she absorbed the acute pain on my left kidney. We were in her kitchen, standing, her hand went straight there where the pain was. A fraction of a second and the pain was gone, never so fast too fast, almost impossible to grasp, to accept. Moving away towards the sitting room, pale when she came back, with a stiff arm, the one that had been hovering away my pain. She could no longer move it.

It took a while to relieve the shock and have her precious arm perfectly moving again. How could she protect herself while so generously open to taking the disease away from me? Never before nor after was there such an evident physical transfer.

Veronica once again, as an indifferent mentor, passed on to me as if a breeze a book, a consolatory one by Ryke Geerd Hamer, Introduction to a new medicine (1). I could not read another book about another alternative approach to cancer. What had intrigued her and me though, was Dr. Hamer's point about the disease's peak. The moment in which the body is completely invaded by disease. According to the German doctor, it is the last resolving phase of the medical conflict causing it. I could not believe it although I wished it was the case.

Explosion of disease, a far more complex explanation made simple. Although I did not want to know any more about its mechanics and causes I would have liked to believe that Dr. Hamer's concept was correct.

Interesting also was the hint about the program of survival a person may enter as a reaction to a conflict, as an immediate solution turning on a flash point, a *focolaio* in the brain, starting in this way a program of survival along which a tumour is born. Have I done that? Was I attached to my tumor, was I actually constantly living with it even when it seemed to have disappeared? Where was it taking me? Which was its plan, its intention, mine?

Tiferet. How peaceful, how comfortable, nothing to explain. The Kabbalah diagram composed of Divine principles, paths and triads, key to comprehending the plan of Existence and our part in it.

Tiferet more than art and ethics, far more, a place of balance and conjunction between earth and sky, of beauty, Divine Beauty (2), not exactly the one well described in the harmonious, homonymus book by John O'Donohue, spotted in the just opened kiosk in Standstead airport, after sunrise during one of my last commuting flights to Rome. Another beauty, O'Donohue; one to be breathed in, on earth, in everyday life.

The more I wanted to be in Tiferet I also longed for divine beauty on earth and I longed for divine beauty on earth because I was in Tiferet.

Let the beauty you love be what you do, (3) Rumi was affirming in his poem. Yes, there I wanted to be, that I wanted to do. Gratitude, enchantment, blessing glimpses of, as if, I were there, but not yet, on my way to, until when? And yes, aware with the Sufi poet again, of the *thousand ways to kneel and kiss the ground.(4)* Poetry, beauty. Kneel and kiss the ground. Honoring. The Sacred.

As for my healer, she could cure my pathologies, no doubt, but, after so much time I was still unable to talk to her about my deep concerns. She was an instrument 'del Signore'. Of God, full stop. She could not agree that we all are instruments of God, that anything, even scientific research is so, even cancer, anything is an instrument and opportunity for us to understand, develop, grow, manifest. There was 'il Signore' with "Dancing with the Stars" and discredit for the work of the mind, for the efforts to understand the causes, to explain life.

If this attitude had been positive as a clean paper on our first approach, after pages of tightly written words, her stubborn denial of anything else but her power above and beyond any other endeavour, skill, gift or activity, was narrowing her potential in my eyes and limiting it in its blind onesidness. Like the one of doctors, not open to anything but their protocols.

All this was making me feel disoriented. Her entity was helping me but was also bossing me around. Her treatments were excellent but I wanted to come out of them. At this later stage the clock on the wall opposite the settee where I placed myself during her treatments had stopped. More precisely the minute hand continued to move but the hour was still, fixed between six and seven. I was stuck, time was passing and I was not going anywhere, not moving forward, not evolving, not progressing, trapped, too dependent on her, less aware than I used to be, less responsible for my health and ability to heal myself; less committed to my own health. She had pulled me more than once out of a disease crisis, but that process was coming to an end.

If you want to obtain a true healing you have to individuate what is governing the spirits, learn how to see them . . . hunt them and become strong enough to defeat them. (5) Wasn't I becoming weaker instead? Hadn't I become dependent on my healer as others had on allopathic medicine? Where had Blanche de force gone? Wasn't I stuck in Rome because of the fear of being invaded by cancer and not having her around and ready to help me? I was becoming aware of an addiction, almost an attachment to the disease, by being less and less at ease, less and less in control of my strength which I'd given up to her. And she so removed so far away from interacting, confronting herself, sharing experiences, exploring the unknown, the unsaid the orthodoxically unaccepted, which was precisely what she was doing.

My shaman was catholic. A contradiction. Perfect. I could not project my way of seeing on her. I was the one who needed logo, I needed to find a logic, to unveil. I needed to be with those, the contemporary, whatever this might mean: the linkers, the breakers of barriers, the holistic, the whole exploring and searching ones. It was like coming out of a head injury, of a deep coma. I knew, I had known, I was remembering, not only words, but ways, of being.

The complex and enlightening research of Candace Perth was more vivid then ever, She as perfectly and essentially described in Deepack Chopra's words, *has provided evidence of the biochemical basis for awareness and consciousness, validating what Eastern philosophers, shamans, rishis, and alternative practitioners have known and practised for centuries. The* Body is not a mindless machine, the body and mind are one. (6)

The reasons of my fascination with her work were equally utterly synthesized by Chopras' words: *in exploring how the mind, spirit, and the emotions are unified with the physical body in one intelligent system . . . , Candace has taken a giant step towards shattering some cherished beliefs held sacred by Western scientists for more than two centuries. Her pioneering research has demonstrated how our internal chemicals, the neuropetides and their receptors, are the actual biological underpinning of our awareness, manifesting themselves as our emotions, beliefs, and expectations, and profoundly influencing how we respond to and experience the world.(7)*

I was feeling well once again thanks to my healer's treatments, but both of us had realized that she could not get to the root of the disease, it clung too deeply to the chest. Too far I had also gone without any medical treatment; nor could I imagine how to face any oncologist. There was a need to balance my experience, to be able to read it to spell out what had happened, what was going on, as if coming out of a cage of mystery which nobody could understand but only accept, as an act of faith, as if it had all been just my fantasy. It wasn't so. It had been a process, a scientific experience of transmutation of coming out of a cocoon. She had been an instrument, an angel, a companion for part of my journey.

Fall 2009. A new shared and luminous home. Not alone, not yet. Lil, the young healer, was practising in Rome once a week. Her daughter, Desiré, was born. Quite a contrast with me, Undesired.

Understanding the speech of my energy, of my past and my future, she started her treatments aiming to modify my vibrations. "We need to find the lock to open the door", she once said, "we shall make it, we need to go deep down to the basic block, then you will be free". From breast we moved to mother. Although previously analysed, with Lil it was like going through a speedy summary, a cause-effect résumé, a very fast journey through the emotions: lack of affection, of love, a now dissolved family, the unhappy ending of a profound love story, the inability to bring to fruition my creations, all wounds to my individuality and feminine side. I was refusing this then and its energetic source or spring, as Lil had defined it, was feeding the tumour.

She was still always dressed in white and I usually wore black. Not all the time. I loved colours and was an expert on nuanced combinations, but for some reason the days of her treatment always ended up being wearing black ones. "Get rid of black" she was inviting me "as well as all the old clothes that accompanied you through all the phases of the disease".

She brought me to a level where, not only did I understand, but also felt that I could make it. She was flexible, open and acute. Soon we started playing - visualisations and intuitive travels. The heaviness of the Roman catholic church and its suffocating, claustrophobic burden with my previous healer's ring standing out as the one of an ecclesiastic. Had she been one of them? The ring she currently wore on the fourth finger of her left hand had appeared as if mounted with a huge precious gem. Had I been feeling this hierarchy, subduing myself to it? I could have been. I was feeling so much rejection to the Church set up but why? Having been so affectionate I came to feel squashed by my catholic healer at the same time. Was the essence of the ring that I was honouring without ever having been myself? Except for my dependence and weakness? Except for my going to her as in pilgrimage, with all the humility of someone who longs to be saved?

I needed to go back to her vibrations and so I visited her, noticing not only how small her ring was but how much larger was the one I was wearing. Mine overshadowed hers in dimension and features. What was going on then? What projection had I created by accepting the miracle and the imposition?

Meanwhile my computer had broken down, no way to restore it and recuperate its files. A new one was needed. I needed to set up my system again, to reprogram myself, my mindset. My chest open, I felt less oppressed, the Church, the Roman Catholic one, its heaviness, my running away from it, its fire, I do not know, its punishment, I fear it, a respect out of fear, would I be killed once again? Is this the reason I was almost expecting my healer was giving me life, was giving life back to me?

Breathing out as much as I could my healer appeared as a small little girl. What was her involvement, what had she done to me? What have I done or not done to her. The little ring was just a tiny precious one, for her, for her family history, no more projection on my part, no more dependency, no more inability to spell out what I thought and felt.

Regular meetings with Lil. Enjoying channelling, travelling to inner places, metaphors for being. Until one day when, lying down on her massage bed, while receiving her energy treatment, I felt an L shaped form inside my body: starting from the right breast it went down across my belly, ending on the left side of the navel. "Hai visto qualcosa" she asked? "Have you seen something?" We had both become aware of the same shape that for her was a luminous one, "like an animal's thick curved leash", she said and for me it was something undefined inside my body, like a scythe connected to a short rod. A sickle.

"Better you have a check up" were her, not immediate, words. "I will". "Do please so we shall know if you are healed or not". I knew I wasn't and also knew that something more radical was necessary to finish off the old story. I was still a heretic, behaving without believing, as an ordinary believer.

Where had that part of me gone? Where was the warrior for truth, the clear loving fearless creature? When had I prevented myself from being so? Adapting homologating, apparently, in the form if not in the essence. Refusing medicalized birth, refusing medicalized treatments, chemotherapy, surgical intervention and ending up as a powerless victim rather than an objectively powerfully choosing person? Why was I hiding my courage, why was I being so different by detaching myself from the masses and ending up not having what everybody else had? Was that a choice? Heresy means choice after all. Was that faith? An impairment of some kind?

Writing, was my joy. I liked it so much. The already started book, this one, entitled 'Living with "C", until then when I decided to get divorced from "C", cancer and transformed the title, first into

'Holding on to destiny'. No other way to explain why, to figure out the journey, the incredible endless steps towards apparently nothing, perceived as an interminable necessary stripping off. My destiny? Don't ask, almost too big a word, Am I refusing it? Am I afraid of it? Why? Why not be myself to the extent of being sick and just be sick, and is being sick almost a justification in order not to be myself? And what if I have never been sick, if it has all been my invention, my excuse, my game in order to sit aside and watch the world? Not to be an interpreter and have all the time to observe and criticize, and to improve the world in my mind? Imagine it as it could be? I had made a few attempts, though. I did get dirty, I dared, but how about the heretic? Where had she gone? Hiding her position, her beliefs silently, living them to death. Dying herself out in silence rather than being sent to death because of her words or actions.

What a pity, what a waste. "Come on Bianca, Biancaaaa!" Lil was calling me, as if from another planet, or was I still so far away from here? "Where are you? Where have you been?" I was asking and telling myself "Coma is over and you are here now".

"Have you done your diagnostic verifications?" She kept asking again and again. "I will". Had to ask for a referral from my GP first, doctor on vacation, it was summer. Had the GP referral by the end of August 2010. Went for blood tests after thirteen years, as if I had been healthy all that time. As if I hadn't needed any, as if living in a desert in a pre-industrial dimension: Siberia, Africa, in the jungle somewhere. Naïve to the new, fearful of results, innocent and well aware. Dreading the blood not stopping after the removal of the needle. It did stop.

Was that a good enough guarantee of health?

"Have you done your check up?" "Yes, no results yet". It took me more than the necessary days to collect them. Tumour markers - these I was looking for. Spotted immediately with a star. 147 - normal value 1.5.

So, it had spread everywhere, all blood contaminated. I became truly scared, called my healer of course and started therapies with her again. Leaving the breast she attacked the ovaries first. I was coughing again from deep down in the belly which was sort of inflated. She had been working on me trying to stem the deluge. A lump along the line of the navel was scaring her and me. It was inserted deep down close to the upper part of the colon. It was rising up when she laid her hand over it and I could measure its unbearable dimensions. The left side of the sickle was 3.5 cm thick and almost 7cm wide and attached to the umbilical chord which had become a stiff tube, connected to the navel. The mass was unchanging despite my healer's treatments. She was irritated and, I could see from her face, very concerned and hopeless, for the first time, as if she could not but surrender.

There was also water, according to her, the big lump was immersed in water. My belly was full of water. What are we doing now? The cancer root of the breast was steadfast to the chest. The lump in the belly was irreducible and what was more important was the question of its nature. What was it?

Nicola was nice and was a radiologist. Frau, a young colleague of mine with Austrian mother and father native of the island of Ischia, told me about him, because his wife was pregnant and wanted to read my book on Birth Places. Frau had also just had an abdomen x-ray and surgical intervention.

Should I maybe go for something similar? "Well Frau, can I book a body scan with your friend?" I was desperately coughing with my 147 tumour markers value secret, constantly on the back of my mind.

She accompanied me, protected and looked after me. The scan report was quite straightforward: pleuric leaking, peritoneal pouring, *centimetric calcific* lymph node in peritoneal area. Something wrong with the right breast and with a particular vertebra. A planned visit to the emergency of a well known hospital would have been the next step to analyse pleuric liquid and the lungs.

Frau accompanied me there as well. Early morning. 7.30 registration and then, while she remained in the reception hall, I followed the path of all the emergency patients. Having entered a long corridor, after a couple of wide rooms I felt suffocated. I carried on and the more I proceeded the worse I felt. Having tried to call my accompanying friend and realizing that there was no field, I went back and let her know that we would not be able to communicate as agreed.

I could not even stay in the reception room, I needed to breath fresh air. Once outside I burst into an unexpected reaction. "I will never get out of there, it is like being in a concentration camp, you enter it and you will never come back". "Calm down" Frau was saying, "No it is like a concentration camp", "Blanche please, please". I did not want to go back. My heart was in pain, I was desperate and lost. It was like going into a no return and no exit tunnel.

What she said to convince me, I don't remember. It was clear that I had to understand how foolish my behaviour was, but it had been compulsory, I could not have avoided it. Having returned to the emergency ward, I realized that my second telephone number, supplied by a different company, was accessible and I felt less at a loss because of that. At least I could communicate with the outside world.

After the check up, a few days later, I was directed to the Pneumology department and from this to the breast cancer oncology department, just after having had an enlightening and freeing dream: transported by ambulance to a hospital I had been sitting in the waiting room until a door opened and Nazi officers came to take me inside the ward. No more doubts about the analogy in my consciousness. No more wondering about my lifelong fight against institutional medicine, against the medical apparatus altogether.

My name was Monika. I knew this from a regression I had been led into when in London in the early nineties. In this life I tended to write my name with a 'k' rather than a 'c': Bianka was so much more natural to me. As it was natural to consider myself slim and taller than I am, as she was, to the point of buying clothes that were far to big for my size. Monika was Polish, wealthy, intellectual,

Jewish. I have been her at the theatre, discussing with scientists, enjoying meals served in the garden of the vast mansion I was living in, the one of my absent father. Single, androgynous, family- less, the woman I felt being with the totality of my different bodies and contexts in this life of mine.

I was on the ledge of the first floor when I saw, down, in the entry hall, a small group of Nazis coming into my house. In the next shot of the regression, there I was, she, dressed as a German soldier, walking quite fast along a path in the woods. While proceeding, and I can still repeat the gesture, I was removing with the back of my right hand tree branches touching my face. The following shot was of me, bold and naked, laying in a foetal position, on the floor of a grey incinerator, my soul exiting my body and going towards the music of a piano playing far away, high up between clouds in the sky.

Had a white dressed doctor injected anything in my body before entering the gas chamber? Were there in the concentration camp doctors inflicting pains rather than soothing them? I could vomit at that simple thought.

My soul, myself, exiting the body, myself going up, almost towards a magnet, there where the sound was coming from.

> *It (the self) is not born, and It does not die; nor is*
> *it ever that this One having been nonexistent*
> *becomes existent again. This One is birthless,*
> *eternal, undecaying, ancient; It is not killed*
> *when the body is killed. (8)*

In my family, this life, my mother's brother and sister both played the piano; my mother having refused it preferring the accordion, which she could never learn to play, it being "very inappropriate for a *signorina*".

I took piano lessons, my first long lasting relationship was with a young man who played the piano, my "first kiss" boyfriend was a piano player too and my right eye, why was it crying incessantly when listening to Chopin Polonaises? Why was the same eye crying again autonomously on the beach, while I listened to Wanda's dramatic story about her father and his sister in the forties and the circumstances in which the woman disappeared and nobody ever heard anything from her again?

Also in the Prague Jewish cemetery, the same uncontrollable sadness without my being aware of being sad at all. And the tape lent by Paul and Kate, a recorded one with a friend of both of ours, giving a speech on television about Previous lives. I had not been surprised when, the program ended, images continued into the classical black and white funereal setting of stations and masses of deported people. I had taken it as a confirmation message. Did they know? I wondered.

There was no train station in Birkenau, where I died; the tracks stopped opposite the entrance to the women's dormitory shelter: crematorium not far, now hidden behind a wood of lush trees.

Bibliography

1 – Ryke Geer Hamer Summary of New Medicine. Amici di Dirk (August 2000)
2 – Divine Beauty The Invisible Embrace John O'Donohue Bantam Books 2003
3 – Jalal Al'Din Rumi – The Book of Love - Poems of Ecstasy and Longing. Coleman Barks (2003).
4 – ibidem
5 – The She-Shaman, Italian title for Entering the Circle: A Russian Psychiatrist's Journey into Siberian Shamanism Olga Kharitidi Gloria Press; 1st edition October 1995
6 – Dipack Chopra in Dipack Chopra in Candace Perth Molecules of emotion The science behind Mind-Body Medicine Simon & Schuster; first edition September 1997
7 – ibidem
8 – Baghavad Gita -Gita Ch.2 Verse 20

CHAPTER 9

CHEMICALLY REMOVING THE LAST RESISTANCES TO LIFE: CHEMOTHERAPY AS REDEEMER

T HE HEAD OF THE Oncology Department was a lady; a breast cancer patient herself of years ago. Women in the waiting room seemed to worship her, so evidently positive, her dedication, her commitment, her indefatigable presence and long hours, as many as were needed.

Her coat hung somehow on the wall of her consulting room. A colleague I would say.

Where shall we start from now? Impossible to explain the medical path.

Diagnosis on 1997. No documents. Lost. The hospital has lost them.

"You can retrieve them". "Yes, I tried but they cannot be found". They were lost in the head of the Anaesthesiology department's office, between papers, underneath papers. I did not say this or that, then he moved hospitals and who knows where my medical records ended up. Lost as if I had never been diagnosed with cancer, as if it had all been my invention, except for a card, a terminally ill patient's card issued after the blood tests before the mastectomy which I never had either. At least there was a document, a proof, a record. Of what? Infiltrating Carcinoma of the breast, the lady oncologist deduced, exactly what I could recall.

"What have you done since 1997?" "Intravenous Vitamin C", this was the only pseudo orthodox non orthodox therapy, with a label, a chemical that could be objectively identified.

"Posso picchiarla?" "Can I beat you up?" were her words while promptly recording my unwillingness to follow traditional therapies. I could see how professionally committed she was and felt and understood all her disappointment for what, according to her, "an intelligent woman had done to herself"

There I was in between the two extremes of right and left brain approaches: the orthodox medical protocol for which I would have been 'experiment' or 'case' number xxx and the orthodox *'via del Signore'* whose ways, as the Bible says, are infinite. So infinite for Science to be tending to zero as accountability

While the lady oncologist was programming further exams in view of chemotherapy, my healer was calling and pressing me to go to her for treatments, 'doctors will kill you', reminding me that *farmaka* in ancient Greek means poisons.

Indeed, at this point I needed a poison, poison to kill you "C"- to get rid of you once for good. The inner work was done, the challenge I gave to myself fulfilled, a sword was needed, a violent stab, not even a back one. Almost hoping for it, *you* were ready, to surrender, you were almost begging to finish you off. You have been around, on and off, for too long. No gentle means but sacrifice, blood for freedom, almost for a celebration, the accomplishment of a task. Mine, yours.

> *Would you believe it Ariadne?*
> *the Minotaur hardly put up a fight (1)*

Theseus words at the end of the House of Asterion chapter in Louis Borges Aleph, a coded sentence between myself and Daniel, now sounded very appropriate to "C".

While aware of the prison condition caused by the pattern motivator of my past memories, I was imagining it prisoner in the door-less maze of my body. A *monster,* like the Minotaur, *scaring people who were praying, prostrating, climbing up to the stylobate of a temple, gathering stones* when seeing it.

A monster, according to the Latin American poet, waiting for his redeemer who would come one day.

Invaded, quite rightly. Chemotherapy as a way to heal myself by helping "C" to die. So convinced so sure and yet so pulled back for seconds, shall I trust, shall I ask other doctors other specialists? Nothing else needs to be done, the coral answer. Chemotherapy first and, being hormone receptive, hormone therapy afterwards. Back to step one of 13 years before.

Same note, but on a different octave

"Si affida?" "Would you entrust yourself to us?" was the oncologist's question. No choice, like the life preserver used by Dad after having done the most he could to rescue others on his battleship, "Roma", that had been broken into two parts by German bombs on the day after the September 8th 1943 armistice between Italy and the Anglo American Allies at the end of world war two. One of the 1,849 people on board the 240 meter long 34 meter wide boat, one of the last to leave it while sinking, one of the 596 who survived by throwing himself into the sea wearing one of the last life preservers on the deck already covered by water.

Jumping with it into the sea, without knowing how to swim, he first could move away from the boat thanks to the wind and some movements on his part, as he explained in a published interview. Half of the ship kneeled over and feeling he would be knocked away, he closed his eyes. Instead, and these are his words, "I was hit by the shifted mass of water, I started to swim until I could see the light".

It was thanks to the wind again that he reached a float from which he could see his ship sinking and from where he was collected by a rifleman.

Gigantic boat sinking and, trusting life, as he said, he himself emerging.

"Mi affido". "I am entrusting myself to you", I confirmed, silently adding: you are now my life preserve.

"Dobbiamo dargli una botta". "We need to hit it" were the lady doctor's words in relation to the chosen type of therapy. We were attuned, violence was necessary, required as I had to explain this to all my healthy cells. Were there any? We needed to bear it, we needed to support the attacks, to be all together hand in hand, almost singing like children in a chorus, while bearing the bombs for their higher purpose.

The nurse had left after completing her procedures to introduce the chemotherapy cocktail into my body by inserting a needle on the outstretched hollow of my left arm. I avoided seeing what she was doing by turning my head to the opposite side and accepting what she did without even looking at it when a bandage was placed on my skin and over the needle to keep it firm. I did not want to see but I could feel something coming from there abouts. A liquid? Caressing my skin. Possibly. I had to look at it, something was overflowing precisely there, where the needle had been inserted. It was my blood pouring out of a small open lid at the top of the pale blue plastic two-way butterfly, at the intersection between the needle in the vein and the thin transparent pipe linked to the bottle, hanging with other transparent plastic bags from the nearby stand. Oh no, are they rejecting the cure? was my first thought. I hoped to have been clear. It is your repulsion, 'yours' meaning 'of you, cells of mine', preventing the liquid to flow in and is the power of your non acceptance driving my own blood out through the second outlet?

Faulty valve was the nurse's comment. "It doesn't happen very often". As a matter of fact what had become the outlet was there to be used as a second inlet.

Removed the needle with the butterfly I simply hoped that you, cells, would not blow out the next one as well. Perfect. Inserted in the right arm flat hollow the new butterfly landed peacefully and diligently started to accomplish its task. No blood spots on the white bandages. All perfectly clean and sterile while flames started to raise from my cheeks up to the fore head. Nurse bell pushed again. With her doctors rushed into the room. Allergy. With the blushing, slight breathing problems: inlet speed decreased, oxygen mask over my mouth. And what's next? While the liquid was very slowly and gently now pouring in I started to wonder if my cells could possibly accept its intrusion at a more reasonable pace. I left after everybody else that day, feeling that the aggression of the bombing at least had been gentle.

Of course I had telephoned first and then placed an order with Ainsworth. *Chemo mix* was on its way. Delays in the UK mail services and my determination to speed up the beginning of the treatment left me without remedies on the first go. Their beneficial effect on the following ones were therefore even more appreciated. They have been my truly nursing companions and allies. They relieved me from most of the expected side effects except for hair falling. I had been warned about that, no way to keep it with *Docetaxel* (3). Locks of hair started to fall out around the 20th day from the first chemo and the true pain was not to be able to shave it off as soon as it started to weaken as friends were suggesting. Shaving would have brought me back to the concentration camp, to the piles of curly and non curly hair in the large container of the Alain Resnais film, "Night and Fog". Masses of light hair, a greater volume than the one of thousands of pairs of glasses, stored in the rather impressive show case in Auschwitz.

While taking me to a beautician for redrawing the eyebrows that would soon fall off too, Serena seduced me into a slow motion hair cut carried out ironically without my being able to watch myself in whatsoever mirror. Sitting next to the wash basin in her bathroom. "Ma quanti capelli hai!" "Look at you, you have so much hair!" "Bugia", "Lie". It took almost half an hour as if I were a little girl to be slowly drawn into drinking a bitter syrup blended into a huge glass of diluted maple juice. It was finally done, maybe she ended earlier than I could see the outcome, but she kept me quiet, I realize it now, preparing me for the view.

Thank you, Serena, if my mind or my skin did not shiver back.

My eyes, huge on the newly bold head, with the following chemo injections, progressively started to change, becoming smaller, red, without expression, or at least with a fish-like expression I could not grasp. Eye lashes disappeared and tears emerged. I had surrendered to chemo, which was working in both ways, destroying in both ways. After the third cocktail the needle could not enter the vein any longer. Luckily, not having gone through surgical intervention, I could offer the other arm, yes, literally as the other cheek, scared for the same consequences that I have then been informed, under request, how to counteract. A cream was enough, just after each injection, massaging the inlet point and the involved vein. Yes, but why wasn't it written, for our own sake, on the wall opposite our Day Hospital beds? The crucified Son was there instead, but no insight from the Holy Spirit about what to do and not to do to help ourselves. Meant to sacrifice? Certainly there to resurrect.

No hints about the consequences of *Zometa* either. Another chemical targeting bone cancer and producing, as side effect, 'only' up to the 10% of cases! and 'only' after years of therapy – how many?, necrosis of the lower jaw. Teeth falling, irremediably, with the side effects of the chemical lasting ten years after the last injection. *Tamoxiphene* was also around, with the side effects I had heard of, mostly replaced by another chemical, produced by the same Italian pharmaceutical company of *Zometa*. Intakes to be monitored because of some potential outcome, plus bone pain.

Nothing new then, interesting for me that I was there, like everybody else, exposed to procedures that I had vehemently avoided all along. There was the fantastic opportunity of having all treatments for free and expensive *farmaka* bought for a few Euros. Amazing for me who was used to paying entirely for my different complementary cures. Two Euros was the cost of the powerful injection meant to regenerate my white blood cells whose value were going down below zero after each chemo treatment. Its effects were the most difficult part of the therapy for me to bear because of the sudden lack of power in the spinal chord becoming weak and difficult to remain erect. The mind was also empty and kept empty to let the rest get on with its job.

I wanted to diligently fulfil the task and I had been fortunate enough to be able to be alone as much as possible not to do and do whatever my body was suggesting.

Was the financial relief good or bad? Wasn't it producing a care free and light hearted overconsumption of *farmaka*, often one antidote to the other? They seemed to work though, miraculously I would say in the case of the fast white blood cells reproduction, but, yes, my buts, why not offer as well less damaging products for the famous building up of the never enough mentioned immune system for instance? And why not teach at school about the physiology of our body, its link with our mind and emotions? Would this have been interfering with hidden agendas of religious matters and corporations interest?

There almost as spectator, this time yes, allowed role, deeply experiencing, fully there, observing the previously unaccepted, taking it for granted in its craziness and helpfulness, this is the way the world goes. The good thing is that I can be helped here, only here, now. The accomplishment was twofold: acceptance of a human condition I had been constantly trying to run away from, and consequent acceptance of myself by others; brothers, relatives and a few colleagues with whom a shared vocabulary for the disease cure was finally found, and consequently, for some of them, even the original diagnosis had been acknowledged.

The healing was vast. After a life of existential searching the existential conciliation was happening through the ordinary, right or wrong it might have been according to holistic principles.

The Minotaur could not wait to be freed. The physical monster in me was on its way to be knocked off and my energies, the blocks maintaining me within my maze, were dissolved. Yes, I had approached the allopathic cure the other way round. Rather than doing the chemo and remove the lump first, and explore all alternative cures I wanted, afterwards, as had been suggested from the beginning, I did the chemo at the closing of the wide-ranging process. Rather stupid on my part I have been discretely told.

Paradoxically I had done it instead the right way. The other way round is the mechanical one from the point of view of the physical body.

I followed the needs of my soul. How could I have explained this when I did not know it myself? Where is the book and by whom is the sentence carefully written by myself so many years ago on its second page: *"you are asking whether the body has a soul? No, it is the soul that has a body"*. The other way round.

Flying towards the clouds, experiencing vividly the painless exit from my body, a natural passage towards a musical freedom. Armeno, were you there, I wonder, waiting for me? I do not remember. Will you be there when I will be ready then?

It happened. To me like to everybody else. It does not matter now my concern for the liquid, my concern for the lump in the peritoneal area. They were there and are not any more. I was coughing and I am not any more. The how is not an issue here. Here is the conclusion of the why. A technical matter, escaping my knowledge and understanding, monitored with my feelings and the capabilities of my body. Up until here yes, I can do, it can be done, it has been necessary, unavoidable.

The sort of partnership I had created to keep myself apart, in the door-less maze of the world, had come to an end. What if I can not make it now? What if . . . but can you imagine, can you believe it as possible? Even if I die, now, I am safe, reconnected to the starting point, at least of this life. I am ready for anything, but I know I shall survive and I shall live.

The congested unlocked, chemotherapy necessary to unwind chemically, a physical and chemical washing away of rusted memories in my veins, arteries, a purification through disinfestation. Weed killer, as in grass field or over fruit trees and vines. Suffocating leaves, suffocating grass blades and suffocating new tender infant grapes and all pain forgotten after the first cleansing rain.

I at the centre of life's purpose in the universal order of becoming.

Biography

1 – The Aleph and Other Stories Penguin Classics 2004
2 – ibidem
3 – *Docetaxel* is an anti-mitotic chemotherapy medication (that is, it interferes with cell division; http://en.wikipedia.org/wiki/Docetaxel

EPILOGUE

AND THE UNVEILING OF
THE KARMIC KNOT

THE OBSESSIVE DEDICATION TO the different phases
and approaches to my sickness, almost an indulgence lasted
fourteen years, has been the only pace my awakening path could
keep up with.

It has been a deepening and broadening process that has strengthened
my awareness of body mind and soul as a whole and has allowed me
to experience both destiny and healing, the former as the continuous
natural evolution of my consciousness within the creative purpose of
the Universe, the latter as alignment of myself with Its all embracing
timelessness in which past present and future coexist.

As if, by a new suddenly established chemical bonds, a life long
turmoil has come to an end and I feel as if it has all been a matter of
fuss about nothing. Immersed in a limitless time, I start to see my
experience in its transformational essence, thus in the qualitative
shift from a before to an after that are now unity and completeness
and that can be differentiated in time and space only from the point
of view of my mind. As matter of fact they are both joined in a
continuity, which is outside and inside myself.

While lacking the language to express this existential change, I am feeling the privilege of the overwhelming experience and I am smiling to cancer, to all the approaches and struggle I have been through, to chemotherapy as well and the 'the ones' I have been, to the blindness of being such a pretentious human creature longing to understand and being totally thick headed in regard to the means of getting 'there', from the beginning, through a reincarnation therapy for instance, since it is the outcome of a tuning in with previous lives experiences that has revealed itself to be so effective at the very end of the journey.

Would that all have been different had I done hypnotic regression on the first place? I had been told about it, I had read and informed myself on those theories, experienced a previous life through meditation and yet the knowledge and the experience had been running over me for decades as if they were the water of a cascading fountain skimming over a marble statue.

The wounds were too big, now I know, so were the grief, the guilt and the pride.

Up until the very end, the process had simply been a pilgrimage of progressive defoliation, a cleansing towards the initiation to wholeness and continuity that have been the natural consequence of important flashes into a specific previous life experience. By dissolving the blockages associated with the wounds of such a particular existence in Renaissance times, a crucial shift has taken place, turning a steady and persistent attitude into the unpredictable one I had been looking for since aeons.

The hints into that specific life, acknowledged during a session purposely booked with a Karmic astrologer while recovering, have contributed to allow it to stand out and regain its identity, distinguish itself from my present one, thus disentangle itself from the inextricable mesh very much alike the blurred image appearing on a screen when few slides are packed in the projector's slot. Precisely as the indistinct projected image, summary of the individual pictures jammed together, vanishes when the slides are inserted one by one, the inextricable mesh, summary of my concealed and intermingled lives, had vanished after having faced the more painful episodes of that specific one.

Once the superimposition of those particular past experiences had vanished, my identification with them has dissolved into a calm cosmic indifference, allowing me to perceive and reconnect at once with the essence of Patience dans l'Azure (1), the Patience in the Azur, chosen by the Canadian astrophysic, and poet, Hubert Reeves as title of his book describing the infinite calmness of the evolving cosmos.

I can not but be immensely grateful to the drive towards being loyal to a truth I could not formulate and for having carried to the end, thus to a new beginning, the paradox of a nature incessantly needing the mind to make sense of evidences by monitoring them with feelings and intuition. A two ways of approaching reality, a critical and an intuitive one, the former related to a rebellious and intolerant nature, the latter to the innocent way of the heart.

Now that I am not any longer held back by the past while holding on to destiny, the former pulling backward and the latter seemingly pulling forward, not any more teared off, distraught and almost stretched as I had been for decades between the two, the disease is not an issue any more, because the healing has taken place there, where the dis-easiness was coming from.

Killed because of my emotions as if I could not allow myself what I liked and was giving me pleasure. The crucial drama I have been held back by relates to a life in the XV-XVI century when, in order to maintain the family inheritance in the hands of my brothers, I have been exiled, without call, to a convent, whose peace, silence, chants, together with the privilege of being able to study with no concern for the practicalities of everyday life, are between the positive memories corresponding to the qualities and activities I still naturally take for granted and enjoy.

While carrying out a life I did not choose but did not dislike, I entered a passionate love affair and became pregnant. In a monastery, where even breasts were bandaged up in order for the most obvious sexual connotation to be disguised, pregnancy had been a nightmare, despite the wide dresses favouring the shapelessness hiding the scandal of the unequivocal contours of the sin of love manifesting, in that specific context, the outstanding expression of a love for sinning. I did gave birth to a girl and I can recall breast feeding my little one until the moment she has been taken away from me.

The subsequent years in jail have been lonely dark and humiliating. Guilt-filled and prevented from life, thus from the joy and happiness of sharing the love I so very well knew about, deprived of my creature and abandoned by the man attracted to my body but to whom status and reputation were dearer than myself, I ended the inflicted punishment with the confession of my sin. The admission was drawn out by the inquisition court after subjecting me to torture and before giving the order to finish me off with poison. Was that genuinely meant for the good of my soul in order to save it through the annihilation of the sinful flesh?

As a matter of fact the declaration drawn out in order to give me the illusion to be forgiven for the so called 'sin' and die in peace had not erased the rebellion against institutional power, dogmas, women and children exploitation, chauvinistic roles, social discrimination, hypocrisy, lies and fabrication nor the intolerance for a not chosen life. It has not even wiped off the conviction of not being allowed to have what was giving me pleasure, even worse, of loosing my life if I would have dared to. Keeping myself well away from family and choosing impossible partners or keeping them at a safe distance, have also been my signal of not being available.

No prince's kiss could have *"unknotted the knot of my heart"* (2) and give me the joy that I firstly needed to regain in myself, independently from events and circumstances. I now also understand of having been carrying the poison in my system and, in a way or another, having been constantly ready to give it back randomly through a kiss.

It is probably M the person who had been aware and could have made me aware of this more than anybody else. While calling me 'Miss Revenge' he was also reproaching me for hiding my body. Disappointed about something I seamed not wanting to grasp he even presented me with a stretching suite wrapping my tin waist and emphasising the good proportions between my hips and breast. I looked adorable in it, but for no reason I had ever chosen that style. My dresses have always been buggy and oversized, now I know, not only because I was still embodying Monika, the Jewish tall woman of the Nazi camp, but mainly to hide or maintain the ambiguity of an undefined shape as if nobody had even to suspect of my pregnancy nor somebody had to choose me for the harmony of my body.

Terrifying, isn't it? I avoid any comment out of compassion because I understand that I needed to go my way to the point of choosing the suffering before this being inflicted on me by others. A curse that needed to be ended and to do so I have taken to the extreme the pattern of having to suffer in order to save myself. My way has been the one of facing the abyss, since, thanks to the wisdom of my soul, I never doubted that "*deep down is the golden ladder leading to the stars*".(3)

Having accepted the challenge of illness and taken the opportunity to experience how "*the big karmic shadow overcomes and overpowers the biological shadow of this life*" (4), I now know, for having experienced it in all my cells, that the purpose of a healing process is the one of clearing the karmic shadow in order to regain what we are thus to honour our nature. This is primarily the message I like to share.

Bibliography

1 – Hubert Reeves Patience dans l'Azur. L'evolution cosmique. Edition du Seuil. 1988
2 – Hugo von Hofmannsthal. La donna senz'ombra. SE Editore, 2008

3 – Hugo von Hofmannsthal. http://www.rodoni.ch/FRAU-OHNE-SCHATTEN/hofmy.html

4 – Thorwald Dethlefesen and Rudiger Dalke- The Healing Power of Illness: Understanding What Your Symptoms Are Telling You – Vega October 2002

www.ingramcontent.com/pod-product-compliance
Lightning Source LLC
Chambersburg PA
CBHW020437290526
45785CB00002B/898